Pressure Ulcers: Recent advances in tissue viability

Also available from Quay Books, MA Healthcare Limited

A–Z Dictionary of Wound Care by Fiona Collins, Sylvie Hampton and Richard J White

Trends in Wound Care, volume I edited by Richard J White

Trends in Wound Care, volume II edited by Richard J White

Trends in Wound Care, volume III edited by Richard J White

Fundamental Aspects of Tissue Viability by Cheryl Dunford and Bridget Günnewicht

Pressure Ulcers: Recent advances in tissue viability

edited by
Michael Clark

Quay Books
MA Healthcare Limited

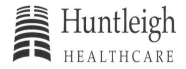

Quay Books Division, MA Healthcare Limited, Jesses Farm, Snow Hill, Dinton, Salisbury, Wiltshire, SP3 5HN

British Library Cataloguing-in-Publication Data
A catalogue record is available for this book

© MA Healthcare Limited 2004
ISBN 1 85642 263 1

Printed by Cromwell Press, Trowbridge

Contents

Section I: Understanding the problem

Section II: Risk factors: facts and fallacies

Section III: Prevention: what works and what doesn't

Section IV: Moving the pressure ulcer debate forward

List of contributors

Hiromi Arao is Assistant Professor, School of Nursing, Oita University, Japan

Yuji Asada is a Doctor, Department of Plastic Surgery, Kansai Rosai Hospital, Japan

Dan Bader, Department of Engineering and the Interdisciplinary Research Centre in Biomedical Materials, Queen Mary and Westfield College, University of London, London

Maureen Benbow is Clinical Nurse Specialist, Tissue Viability, Leighton Hospitral

Gerry Bennett was Professor of Geriatric Medicine, Royal London Hospital, Mile End, London

Gerrie Bours, University of Maastricht, Department of Nursing Science, the Netherlands. She is Chair of the EPUAP Pressure Ulcer Prevalence Project Steering Group

Martyn Butcher is Clinical Nurse Specialist, Tissue Viability, Derriford Hospital, Plymouth

Michael Clark is Senior Research Fellow, Wound Healing Research Unit, University of Wales College of Medicine, Cardiff

Carol Dealey is Research Fellow, Nursing and Therapy Research Unit, University of Birmingham and University Hospital Birmingham NHS Trust

Tom Defloor is Professor of Nursing Science, based at the University of Gent, Department of Nursing Science, Belgium

Krzys Gebhardt is Clinical Nurse Specialist, Tissue Viability, St George's Hospital, London

Satsue Hagisawa is Professor, School of Nursing, Nagoya City University, Japan

Miles E Maylor is Senior Lecturer in Tissue Viability, University of Glamorgan, Wales

Jill Pell is Consultant in Public Health Medicine, Greater Glasgow Health Board

Shyam VS Rithalia, School of Health Care Professions, University of Salford

Tatsuo Shimada is Professor, School of Nursing, Oita University, Japan

Iain Swain is Consultant Biomedical Engineer, Salisbury Healthcare NHS Trust, Salisbury and Professor of Clinical Engineering, Bournemouth University, Bournemouth

Gail Teasley is Outcomes Research Manager, Williamsburgh, Virginia, USA

Kieran Walsh is Specialist Registrar, Colchester General Hospital, Colchester

Lynne Watret is Tissue Viability Nurse, North Glasgow Hospitals University NHS Trust

Susan Williams is Mary Thomson Research Fellow, Greater Glasgow NHS Board

Jim Zoller is Project Statistician, Charleston, SC, USA

Foreword

A book edited by Michael Clark can be bought without hesitation. Michael is at present, to the best of my knowledge, one of the most experienced people in the field of pressure ulcers.

I have read this book and, as expected, found it excellent. The content is laid out in a logical order. It starts with a description of what the problem is all about: the progress that has been made in the last ten years in pressure ulcer management and the impact of the problem across Europe. This last question is dealt with by looking at both prevalence and incidence. Recently, there was some debate in the European Pressure Ulcer Advisory Panel (EPUAP) about the method of recording pressure ulcer occurrence that should be used. Prevalence seemed to be easy in early studies and provides rough determinations of the magnitude, while incidence is more precise and able to identify the causative factors and should be used in programs destined to reduce the occurrence of pressure ulcers. The second section considers risk factors dealing with basic investigations into the microscopic anatomy of the skin, along with the issue of the recording and interpretation of interface pressure measurements. The third section on prevention covers aspects of turning the patient as well as support surfaces and their technology. The final section is about the way studies should be conducted in pressure ulcer care and concludes with a chapter to which Gerry Bennett, who died only some months ago, contributed. For those who knew and worked with Gerry, it is typical that this chapter does not depict his personal experiences on how to use surfaces or which type of dressing to apply, but deals with the role of abuse and neglect and how the GP should be involved. It is not surprising that Michael decided to end this book with a chapter from Gerry for we both valued, and learned from his contribution to the topic of pressure ulcers.

This book, written by a group of excellent researchers, will contribute greatly to the literature already available on pressure ulcers. Read it carefully, it is worth it.

Jeen RE Haalboom,
Professor of Internal Medicine and former President of the EPUAP
University Hospital Utrecht, the Netherlands
March, 2004

Introduction

Pressure ulcers, their causes, prevention and treatment have in the past few years begun to receive the serious attention they deserve. We now stand at a cusp in our endeavours in pressure ulceration with the future holding out the promise of enhanced understanding of the causes of these wounds along with more rigorous evidence of the effectiveness of the interventions commonly used in the fight against pressure ulcers. This growing body of rigorous evidence builds upon the previous efforts of enthusiastic individuals, drawn from many professional backgrounds and countries that together created such organisations as the Tissue Viability Society in the United Kingdom and the European Pressure Ulcer Advisory Panel (EPUAP). This book seeks to draw from the experience of these pioneers, to reflect upon the growing maturity of today's pressure ulcer research community and to offer tantalising glimpses of what the immediate future may hold.

The individual chapters have been drawn from recent publications within several key sources – the *Journal of Tissue Viability*, the *British Journal of Nursing*, the *British Journal of Health Care Management*, the *EPUAP Review*, and finally *Nursing and Residential Care*. Each chapter has been reviewed by its authors and updated where required. In this way this publication seeks to reflect and consolidate current research themes in pressure ulceration. Obviously, such a publication would be impossible without the support of the editorial teams within each journal and I would like to thank each title for making access available to their original publications. As editor I have limited my role to the offering of key observations upon each chapter — these reflect my own views upon the priorities we face within understanding and managing pressure ulcers.

The book is divided into four main themes: pressure ulcer epidemiology, understanding pressure ulcers, the effectiveness of interventions and a look into the future. These themes well reflect the key issues in pressure ulceration today and it is also without apology that the focus of this book rests upon pressure ulcer prevention. Do not explore this book looking for new insights into wound dressings and local treatments for pressure ulcers — this information is well represented elsewhere! Some years ago the pressure ulcer community in the United Kingdom held to the assertion that 95% of pressure ulcers were preventable. We may quibble over what, if any, science supports such a claim but the message has not lost its force even twenty years after its initial publication. One clear goal today is to understand just how far we can intervene within the myriad pathways that individually and together lead to the genesis of a pressure ulcer. So, this book holds prevention as the ultimately desirable goal and many of the chapters reflect this theme.

It would be wonderful if the publications that together comprise this book represented the very pinnacle of scientific thought and enquiry in pressure ulceration. This is not the case for many of the studies have been selected to illustrate themes; the emerging role of new researchers, the multi-professional nature of pressure ulcer research and the need to co-operate with colleagues both local and world-wide are recurrent issues that emerge within the individual sections. Many of the individual studies (and, in particular, the randomised controlled trials) covered in this book may fail to achieve high marks for their internal quality but that reflects where we are in the field in the early years of the twenty-first century. We must now build upon these controlled trials, improving the quality of our designs, along with our study execution and its subsequent reporting — this is just one of the challenges for the immediate future. For now, the clinical trials reported in this book should be considered to mark important first steps along the way to achieving high quality clinical trials in pressure ulceration.

Let us not look too negatively at the studies done to date; there are lessons to learn but we as a tissue viability community are maturing rapidly. It is this maturation process that this book seeks to highlight — perhaps controversially in places it raises the spectre that we have not been too clever in the past years! The whole question of pressure ulcer occurrence and apparent trends over time is a recurrent issue within the book — for this may well be the single largest gap in our knowledge at this time.

On a personal note, I was surprised to find myself working upon this title — for twenty years in pressure ulceration I held the view that books were of less importance than research communications. However, the preparation of this title allowed me to see that we face enormous opportunities in the coming years: new research funding, a shrinking world, a growing cadre of trained researchers interested in pressure ulcers and a blending of the professional roles and inputs to tissue viability. This book hopefully serves as a watershed between enthusiasm and the emergence of a scientific discipline(s) we may be proud to call tissue viability. For this reason, I am very pleased to have been invited to edit this coming of age publication.

Michael Clark
Senior Research Fellow
Wound Healing Research Unit
University of Wales College of Medicine, Cardiff
February, 2004

Section I:
Understanding the problem

This section initially provides a rapid overview of the most significant advances in pressure ulceration over recent years. This helps set the accelerating pace of interest in pressure ulcers in context and provides a focus for the remainder of the book. Having discussed the environment in which pressure ulcer clinical practice and research exists; two important issues in monitoring pressure ulcer occurrence are introduced — the need for consistent data collection methods and the 'holy grail' of comparable data! Consistent data collection lay at the heart of a recent European pilot project that developed a pressure ulcer prevalence data collection tool and piloted this across twenty-six hospitals in five European countries, highlighting one principle theme in this book: the achievements that can occur when we, in different disciplines and countries come together and share and develop projects collectively. The final chapter in this section well illustrates that risk adjustment or case-mix adjustment of pressure ulcer incidence data does not lie only in the realm of academic research but can, and should be, a powerful tool for clinicians. Working with an audit department in the west of Scotland, local clinicians have been involved in collecting pressure ulcer incidence data and then seeking to adjust this raw data to take account of differences in the characteristics of the surveyed patients, bringing new insights into the scale of the problem of pressure ulcers within the wards that participated in this study. Risk adjustment of pressure ulcer occurrence data is one key step we need to take if our efforts to understand pressure ulceration are to mature fully.

1

Review of advances in pressure ulcer management since 1992

Carol Dealey

This chapter seeks to review the progress in the treatment and prevention of pressure ulcers over the last ten years under the headings of attitudes, politics, research and best practice. It is considered that attitudes have changed and there is a greater awareness of, and interest in, the topic among other healthcare professionals, not just nurses. This may in part be because the topic has risen up the political agenda following studies which have highlighted the numbers of sufferers and the cost of treatment. Unfortunately, there is a scarcity of high quality research to inform practice. Despite these limitations, overall, there has been some progress in preventing and treating pressure ulcers, but there is still a considerable journey ahead.

Attitudes

In 1992, pressure ulcers were seen as very much a nursing problem (Dealey, 1992). Few doctors were interested in the topic and most abdicated any responsibility for it. There was a tendency to deny the existence of pressure ulcers and many nurses claimed that the only pressure ulcers they saw were the ones that came in from elsewhere. Happily, in 2002, there is greater awareness of the problem. More healthcare professionals, including doctors, take an interest in pressure ulcers. Nevertheless, pressure ulcers cannot be described as a glamorous topic and may never attract the interest and the resources needed to reduce drastically their numbers.

Politics

Over the last ten years pressure ulcers have gradually moved up the political agenda, both in the UK and elsewhere. Cynically, it would be easy to say that this is because of the greater awareness of the large numbers of sufferers and the cost to health systems. Certainly, these two issues must both be considered under the banner of politics.

Prevalence

Prevalence surveys have been used to demonstrate the considerable numbers of patients with pressure ulcers, particularly in Europe and in North America. *Figure 1.1* shows the many countries in Europe that have undertaken surveys, demonstrating the widespread interest. This interest has increased since pressure ulcers have become recognized as an indicator of the quality of care (Department of Health [DoH], 1993). Some countries, notably Belgium and the Netherlands, undertake regular national surveys. In the USA, this is done on alternate years. In the UK, there has been less interest in undertaking this type of survey at a national level.

Haalboom *et al* (1997) consider that there have been remarkably similar figures across countries with results showing prevalence rates ranging from 5%–15%. This is supported by the most recently published national survey from the USA which found a prevalence of 14.8% (Amlung *et al*, 2001).

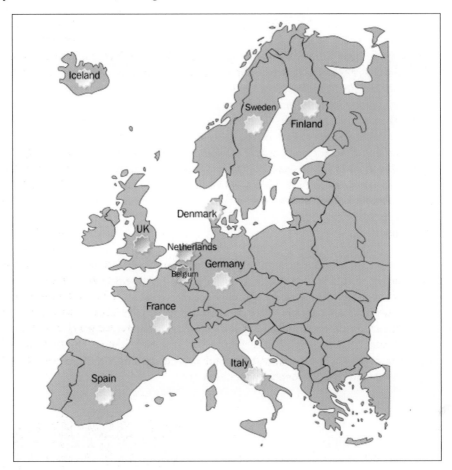

Figure 1.1: A map of Europe showing the countries which have undertaken pressure ulcer prevalence surveys. Orange denotes many surveys

Costs

The considerable amounts of money spent on treating pressure ulcers has attracted political attention. In the USA, it has been estimated that the cost is around $1.3 billion each year (Gallagher, 1997). Recent figures from the Netherlands suggest that the cost of treating pressure ulcers ranges from 1%–6% of the total Dutch healthcare budget (Severens *et al*, 2002). Cost can also be measured in terms of extended length of stay as shown by Allman *et al* (1999) who found that patients with pressure ulcers had a significantly longer length of stay than people without pressure ulcers (30.4 days *vs*

12.8 days). Litigation costs also have to be considered. Tingle (1997) described several legal cases with settlements ranging from £3500–£12500.

Policies

A major turning point in the UK was the publication of the document entitled *Pressure Sores: a Key Quality Indicator* (DoH, 1993). Other documents have followed, including national guidelines from the National Institute for Clinical Excellence (NICE, 2001). Many other countries have developed guidelines for pressure ulcer prevention and management and there are also European Guidelines (European Pressure Ulcer Advisory Panel [EPUAP], 1998). All this serves to demonstrate the increased interest in the topic.

Research

Guidelines are based on research evidence which is graded in order to quantify the strength of evidence to support each statement within the guideline. *Figure 1.2* shows the three grades of evidence used in NICE guidelines and numbers of statements supported by each grade of evidence. It is worrying that the majority of statements are supported by level three evidence.

Systematic reviews of research, such as that undertaken by Gould *et al* (2000), of the impact of nursing interventions on the prevalence and incidence of pressure ulcers, have persistently reported that the research studies are poor methodologically. There is obviously an urgent need to improve the quality of research undertaken in this area.

However, there is some good evidence available as identified by the most recent Cochrane review of beds, mattresses and cushions (Cullum *et al*, 2004). In a survey of twenty-nine randomized controlled trials it was found that there was good evidence of: the effectiveness of high performance foam over standard foam; the effectiveness of pressure relief in the operating theatre; and the effectiveness of both air fluidized and low air loss beds for treating pressure ulcers.

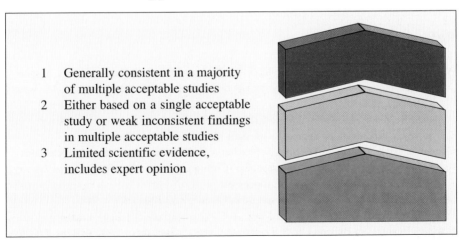

1   Generally consistent in a majority of multiple acceptable studies
2   Either based on a single acceptable study or weak inconsistent findings in multiple acceptable studies
3   Limited scientific evidence, includes expert opinion

Figure 1.2: Levels of evidence in National Institute for Clinical Excellence pressure ulcer guideline

Best practice

It is quite obvious that a great deal of our prevention strategies are dependent on best practice rather than research, which is much the same as it was in 1992. However, there does appear to be a greater consensus of opinion today than there was ten years ago. There is also an awareness of the current research and its limitations.

There are areas where best practice and research evidence diverge, for example, risk calculators. There are currently thirty to forty different risk calculators in use, often with little research involved in their development. There is no evidence to show whether they are any better than clinical judgment (Effective Health Care Bulletin, 1995). Many experts and local policies and guidelines recommend the use of a risk calculator and it is generally seen as good practice to assess the level of risk of patients in this way. It is certainly expected in litigation cases that patients will have had this type of formal assessment.

Conclusion

So, have we moved on over the last ten years? I believe that we have made some good progress, but there is still a long way to go before we have a true understanding of the pathophysiology of pressure ulcers and how they can best be prevented and treated.

Key points

⌘   Pressure ulcers have become recognized as a costly and painful problem.

⌘   The prevalence of pressure ulcers has been found to range from 5–15%.

⌘   There are a number of guidelines available for the prevention and management of pressure ulcers.

⌘   Unfortunately there is limited good quality research available to support these guidelines.

References

Allman RM, Goode PS, Burst N, Bartolucci AA, Thomas DR (1999) Pressure ulcers, hospital complications and disease severity: impact on hospital costs and length of stay. *Adv Wound Care* **12**(1): 22–30

Amlung SR, Miller WL, Bosley LM (2001) The 1999 national pressure ulcer prevalence survey: a benchmarking approach. *Adv Skin Wound Care* **14**(6): 297–301

Cullum N, Deeks J, Sheldon TA, Song F, Fletcher AW (2004) Beds, mattresses and cushions for pressure sore prevention and treatment (Cochrane Review). In: *The Cochrane Library*, Issue 1, John Wiley and Sons Ltd, Chichester

Dealey C (1992) Pressure sores: the result of bad nursing? *Br J Nurs* **1**(15): 748

Department of Health (1993) *Pressure Sores: A Key Quality Indicator*. DoH, London

Effective Health Care Bulletin (1995) The prevention and treatment of pressure sores. *Effective Health Care Bulletin* **2**(1): 1–16

European Pressure Ulcer Advisory Panel (1998) A policy statement on the prevention of pressure ulcers from the European Pressure Ulcer Advisory Panel. *Br J Nurs* **7**(15): 888–90

Gallagher S (1997) Outcomes in clinical practice: pressure ulcer prevalence and incidence studies. *Ostomy and Wound Management* **43**: 28–38

Gould D, James T, Tarpet A, Kelly D, Pattison D, Fox C (2000) Intervention studies to reduce the incidence and prevalence of pressure sores: a literature review. *J Clin Nurs* **9**(2): 163–77

Haalboom JRE, van Everdingen JJE, Cullum N (1997) Incidence, prevalence and classification. In: Parish LC, Witkowski JA, Crissey JT, eds. *The Decubitus Ulcer in Clinical Practice.* Springer Publishing Company, New York: 12–23

National Institute for Clinical Excellence (2001) *Inherited Clinical Guideline: Pressure Ulcer Risk Assessment and Prevention.* NICE, London

Severens JL, Habraken JM, Duivenvoorden S, Frederiks CMA (2002) The cost of illness of pressure ulcers in the Netherlands. *Adv Skin Wound Care* **15**(2): 72–7

Tingle J (1997) Pressure sores: counting the legal cost of nursing neglect. *Br J Nurs* **6**(13): 757–8

2

A pilot study of the prevalence of pressure ulcers in European hospitals

Michael Clark, Tom Defloor and Gerrie Bours

The European Pressure Ulcer Advisory Panel (EPUAP) has conducted a pilot survey of the prevalence of pressure ulcers across a range of hospitals located within five European countries (Belgium, Italy, Portugal, Sweden and the United Kingdom). This report describes the data gathered across all of these countries. A total of 5947 patients were surveyed over the fourteenth and fifteenth of November 2001 (and on the fifth February 2002 when all Swedish data was obtained), and of these 1078 (18.1%) had pressure ulcers. The prevalence of pressure ulcers within each country ranged from 8.3% (Italy) to 22.9% (Sweden).

The anatomical locations most commonly affected by pressure ulcers were the sacrum (in Italy and the UK) and the heels (Belgium, Portugal and Sweden). Of the 1078 patients with a pressure ulcer(s) the greatest number (n=454, 42.1%) experienced non-blanching erythema as their most severe form of pressure damage. However, 143 patients experienced the most severe form of pressure damage (Grade 4 wounds).

The proportion of surveyed patients who received no pressure ulcer preventive interventions ranged from 10.4% (UK) to 92.1% (Italy), with relatively few patients receiving interventions deemed to be fully appropriate (n=265, 4.6%). It should be noted that the pilot study did not recruit a representative sample of hospital sites and so the data presented within this report can not be considered to represent the 'true' picture of the prevalence and characteristics of pressure ulcers across acute care in Europe.

Background

One of the most common measures of the occurrence of pressure ulcers has been their prevalence, defined as the number of people with a pressure ulcer as a proportion of the entire patient population over a defined period of time. Pressure ulcer prevalence has been reported over the years across many countries and many healthcare providers. This measure provides information upon the current numbers of patients with pressure ulcers and the characteristics of their wounds. Measures of prevalence are not suitable for identifying improvements in pressure ulcer occurrence following changes in practice, given that prevalence includes patients admitted to a hospital with established pressure ulcers.

Comparison between these myriad prevalence proportions has been limited by various issues related to the performance of each survey. Among the many confounding issues are:

⌘ **Which patient groups have been surveyed?** Have areas such as maternity where pressure ulcers may be rare been included or excluded?

⌘ **How have pressure ulcers been defined**? Did the survey count areas of non-reactive erythema as a pressure ulcer or were only frank skin breaks counted?

⌘ **How was the data collected?** Was the skin of all patients examined or were the results based on information passed by clinical staff?

These and many other factors effectively preclude any comparison between hospitals, regions and countries. For this reason, the European Pressure Ulcer Advisory Panel (EPUAP) instigated a working group in 2000 to develop and test a methodology which would allow such comparisons to be made. The members of this working group are listed in Appendix 1 at the end of this chapter. Heavily influenced by the work of the research team responsible for the annual Dutch national pressure ulcer survey, the EPUAP working group developed a data collection instrument (shown in Appendix 2 of this chapter) and piloted this instrument across five European countries (Belgium, Italy, Portugal, Sweden and the United Kingdom) over the fourteenth and fifteenth of November 2001 (and the fifth February 2002 when Swedish data was collected). This report provides an overview of the data collected within these five European countries during the pilot survey.

Survey methodology

In each country a national co-ordinator (NC) was appointed from among the ranks of the EPUAP trustees and their work colleagues. The primary roles of the NC were to identify potential hospitals in which data on the prevalence of pressure ulcers would be collected and to facilitate staff within these hospitals to undertake the survey. The goals of the pilot survey were: a) to collect data from approximately 1000 hospital patients within each country and, b) to explore issues related to the implementation of a system for collecting prevalence data that could be used in different countries.

Having identified potential hospitals within each country, research ethics applications covering the performance of the survey were submitted (where each country's regulations required this to be done) and approval for data collection obtained. Over the period of fourteenth and fifteenth November 2001 (and fifth February 2002 in Sweden) the skin of all in-patients staying overnight on the day of the survey was inspected by two nurses; one drawn from the clinical area's staff, while the second formed part of the research team within each participating hospital.

During the survey information was collected upon the presence, anatomical location and severity of pressure ulcers. Each pressure ulcer's severity was assessed using the EPUAP pressure ulcer classification tool (see Appendix 3), while each patient's vulnerability to developing pressure ulcers was assessed using the Braden scale. While the Braden scale allows assessment of skin moisture it does not specifically address continence, and the EPUAP working group also included the continence section of the Norton scale within the data collection instrument. No attempt was made to combine the Braden and continence scores into a single indicator of possible vulnerability to pressure ulcers.

On two selected wards within each hospital, two members of the research team independently inspected the skin of patients to establish the level of agreement between observers. Across all participating countries the level of agreement between observers was very high (for the Braden scale 0.985, for the most severe pressure ulcer 0.963, and for the location with the most severe grade of pressure ulcer 0.934 all of these were significant at a *p* value of < 0.001). All completed forms were copied with the original data sheets returned to a central point for data processing and analysis.

Results

A total of 5947 patients were surveyed across the five countries, of these 1078 (18.1%) had established pressure ulcers. Patients were surveyed across twenty-six hospital sites with 48.2% (*n*=2868) of all patients nursed within teaching hospitals, the remainder within general hospitals (*Table 2.1*). Of the 5947 patients surveyed, 2544 (42.8%) were located in the United Kingdom (drawn from eleven hospitals in England, two in Wales and two in Northern Ireland).

Table 2.1: The number of patients and the number of participating hospitals reported across the five countries that participated within the pilot prevalence study

	University hospital	Patients	Range of patients per centre	General hospital	Patients	Range of patients per centre
Portugal	-	-	-	3	786	154–441
Belgium	1	665	665	1	206	206
UK	4	820	22–567	11	1724	32–347
Sweden	2	613	24–589	1	36	36
Italy	2	770	243–527	1	327	327
Total	**9**	**2868**		**17**	**3079**	

a) Patient demographic information.

The age of the surveyed patients was collected as a series of age ranges (for example, whether the patient was aged between eighty and eighty-nine years) and, as such, it is not possible to calculate the mean age of the surveyed population. *Table 2.2* highlights the age distribution of the surveyed patients with 2921 (49.1%) aged over seventy years old. The age of forty-two (0.7%) subjects was unreported. The mode age range varied by country, for example, in Belgium, most patients surveyed were between forty and forty-nine years old, with over 12% under eighteen years old. Across the other four countries patients tended to be older; mode age range seventy to seventy-nine years (Italy and Portugal) and eighty to eighty-nine years in Sweden and the United Kingdom. Most patients were female (*n*=3088, 52.9%) with the sex of 109 (1.8%) unreported. The percentage of each country's surveyed patients where gender was unreported ranged from 0.9% (Portugal) to 3.6% (Italy). It is important to note that the demographic information presented in this section of the report includes all surveyed patients and not just those with pressure ulcers.

Table 2.2: The age of patients surveyed by country

	Number (percentage) of patients within each age group							
	Under 12 years	12–18 years	19–39 years	40–59 years	60–69 years	70–79 years	80–89 years	>89 years
Portugal	28 (3.6)	9 (1.1)	83 (10.6)	175 (22.3)	165 (21.0)	217 (27.7)	89 (11.4)	18 (2.3)
Belgium	77 (8.9)	19 (2.2)	109 (12.6)	201 (23.2)	155 (17.9)	160 (18.4)	112 (12.9)	35 (4.0)
UK	1 (0)	19 (0.8)	268 (10.6)	400 (15.8)	402 (15.9)	618 (24.4)	628 (24.8)	197 (7.8)
Sweden		3 (0.5)	50 (7.8)	152 (23.6)	104 (16.1)	129 (20.0)	167 (25.9)	39 (6.1)
Italy	42 (3.9)	11 (1.0)	93 (8.6)	187 (17.4)	231 (21.5)	295 (27.4)	176 (16.4)	41 (3.8)
Total	**148 (2.5)**	**61 (1.0)**	**603 (10.2)**	**1115 (18.9)**	**1057 (17.9)**	**1419 (24.0)**	**1172 (19.8)**	**330 (5.6)**

Table 2.3: Distribution of male and female patients by country

Country	Number of male patients	Number of female patients
Belgium	406	445
Italy	556	502
Portugal	417	362
Sweden	312	321
United Kingdom	1059	1458
Total	**2750**	**3088**

There are many different descriptions for the various medical specialities across Europe and in an attempt to make definition consistent across all countries that might use the EPUAP prevalence data collection instrument, generic categories covering medical speciality were constructed. For example, 'acute care/high dependency' would include many surgical wards, while 'chronic care' would include long-term care of the elderly. Based upon these definitions, most of the patients were considered to be acute care/high dependency patients (n=3703, 63.0%) (*Table 2.4*). Only in Portugal did the mode care group differ with most patients surveyed considered to receive chronic care. Despite the unfamiliarity of these definitions the care group was unreported in only 68 (1.1%) cases.

The vulnerability of each patient to developing pressure ulcers was assessed using the Braden scale, this tool similar in structure to the Norton and Waterlow scales, provides a summary score based upon six patient characteristics — their ability to respond to sensory stimuli, the moistness of their skin, their activity, mobility and exposure to shear forces and, finally, their nutritional intake. A Braden score of 16 or below is typically considered to mark a need for preventive interventions to be undertaken to prevent pressure ulcer development.

Typically, the Braden scores recorded for the patients surveyed across the participating European countries ranged from 6 to 23, median score 19. The exceptions to this were; the minimum Braden scores recorded in Portugal and Sweden were 7 and 9 respectively, while the median Braden score recorded in Italy was 21. Based on their Braden scores, 1733 (29.1%) of all surveyed patients were at risk of developing pressure damage (*Table 2.5*). The percentage of patients considered at risk of developing pressure ulcers was highest in Belgium (34.9%) and the United Kingdom (33.2%). The Braden scores of 187 patients were unreported during the surveys. Most unreported Braden scores occurred among the surveyed Italian patients (*n*=85, 7.7%), with the most complete risk assessment data derived in Portugal (missing data *n*=4, 0.5%).

Table 2.4: Location of the patients in each surveyed country by medical age group

	Neurology	Intensive	Chronic care	Acute care/ high dependency
Portugal	145 (18.5)	65 (8.3)	304 (38.8)	270 34.4)
Belgium	149 (17.3)	74 (8.6)	209 (24.3)	427 (49.7)
UK	375 (14.8)	43 (1.7)	456 (18.0)	1653 (65.4)
Sweden	35 (5.5)	32 (5.0)	84 (13.2)	487 (76.3)
Italy	125 (11.7)	55 (5.1)	25 (2.3)	866 (80.9)
Total	**829 (14.1)**	**269 (4.6)**	**1078 (18.3)**	**3703 (63.0)**

b) Vulnerability to pressure ulcer development.

Table 2.5: Vulnerability to developing pressure ulcers by country. Percentages based upon the total number of patients with reported Braden scores (*n*=5760)

Country	Not at risk (Braden score 17+)	% not at risk	At risk (Braden score 16 or lower)	% at risk
Belgium	562	65.1	301	34.9
Italy	783	77.4	229	22.6
Portugal	551	70.5	231	29.5
Sweden	468	76.2	146	23.8
United Kingdom	1663	66.8	826	33.1
Total	**4027**	**69.9**	**1733**	**30.1**

Use of the Braden scale was supplemented by the capture of specific information upon each patient's level of continence using the continence section of the Norton scale. This section offers four possible responses scored from 1 (fully continent) to 4 (doubly incontinent). While inclusion of the continence section of the Norton scale offers more information that may pertain to the current risk of a patient developing pressure ulcers, it may be difficult to complete given a lack of operational definitions — for example, how should an incontinent but catheterised patient be scored? Regardless of these issues, most patients were assessed as being continent (*n*=4417, 75.1%) (*Table 2.6*). Most doubly incontinent patients were found among the Belgian (16.4%) and UK (10.7%) surveyed patients. The continence status of sixty-nine (1.2%) patients was unreported with thirty-eight missing cases within the Italian survey (3.5% of all patients surveyed in Italy).

Across the five countries represented within the survey, 1078 patients were reported to have pressure ulcers, with the overall prevalence by country illustrated in *Figure 2.1*. Three countries (Belgium, Sweden and the United Kingdom) had similar prevalence proportions ranging from 21.1% to 22.9%. The prevalence of pressure ulcers was reported to be lower in both Italy (8.3%) and Portugal (12.5%).

Table 2.6: Reported continence of the surveyed patients by country. Data shows both the absolute numbers of patients and the percentage, shown in parenthesis, within each category

Country	Continent	Occasional incontinence	Urinary incontinence	Double incontinence
Belgium	577 (66.3)	110 (12.6)	40 (4.6)	143 (16.4)
Italy	920 (86.9)	69 (6.5)	38 (3.6)	32 (3.0)
Portugal	601 (76.8)	102 (13.0)	21 (2.7)	59 (7.5)
Sweden	512 (79.6)	60 (9.3)	33 (5.1)	38 (5.9)
United Kingdom	1807 (71.6)	353 (14.0)	93 (3.7)	270 (10.7)
Total	**4417 (75.1)**	**694 (11.8)**	**225 (3.8)**	**542 (9.2)**

c) Number, severity and distribution of encountered pressure ulcers

The 1078 patients with pressure ulcers experienced a total of 1860 pressure ulcers, with the sacrum the commonly affected site ($n=532$, 28.6%). *Figure 2.2* illustrates the anatomical distribution of all encountered pressure ulcers. Almost 88% (1630/1860; 87.6%) of all encountered pressure ulcers were found at one of eleven anatomical locations (*Table 2.7*). Several differences were apparent between the relative distributions of pressure ulcers over body sites. For example, both Italy and the United Kingdom exhibited higher percentages of sacral pressure ulcers compared with the other countries (40.9% and 37.5% respectively of all pressure ulcers reported during the Italian and British surveys were located on the sacrum). Other differences between countries were also evident; for example, the high percentages of ankle and hip pressure ulcers in Sweden and Portugal respectively.

Table 2.7: Anatomical distribution of the pressure ulcers encountered at the most commonly affected body sites by country. Data shows absolute numbers of pressure ulcers and the percentage, shown in parenthesis, within each category. (L/R denotes that the category combines pressure ulcers reported at the left and right body sites)

Location	Belgium	Italy	Portugal	Sweden	United Kingdom	Total
Sacrum	77 (25.6)	54 (40.9)	50 (26.9)	59 (25.3)	292 (37.5)	532
Heel L/R	105 (34.9)	42 (31.9)	63 (33.9)	70 (30.0)	204 (26.2)	484
Ischium L/R	37 (12.2)	10 (7.6)	5 (2.7)	27 (11.6)	107 (13.7)	186
Ankle L/R	11 (3.6)	12 (9.1)	19 (10.2)	57 (24.5)	50 (6.4)	149
Elbow L/R	43 (14.3)	0	13 (6.9)	7 (3.0)	80 (10.3)	143
Hip L/R	28 (9.3)	14 (10.6)	36 (19.3)	13 (5.6)	45 (5.8)	136
Total	**301**	**132**	**186**	**233**	**778**	**1630**

The most severe pressure ulcer was recorded for all patients with pressure ulcers. Typically the most severe pressure ulcer presented as areas of non-blanchable erythema ($n=454$, 42.1% of all patients with pressure ulcers experienced such wounds as their most severe area of pressure damage). The severity and anatomical locations of the most severe pressure ulcer experienced by the surveyed patients are illustrated in

Figures 2.3 and 2.4 respectively. Typically, the sacrum was the body site that experienced the most severe pressure ulcers.

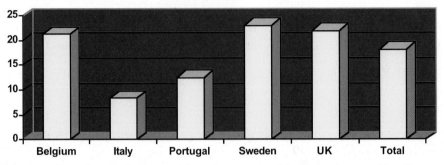

Figure 2.1: Prevalence of pressure ulcers by country. Vertical columns show the percentage of patients with pressure ulcers in each country

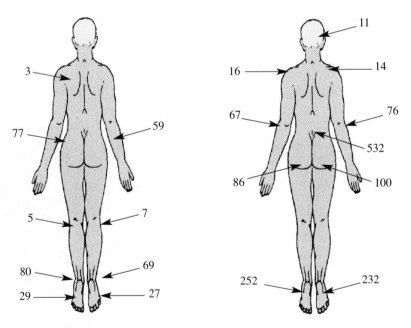

Figure 2.2: Anatomical distribution of pressure ulcers encountered across all patients surveyed. Numbers refer to the number of pressure ulcers at each anatomical site. Pressure ulcers also occurred 118 times at sites not illustrated in the figure

The most severe form of pressure ulcer (Grade 4) occurred in 143 patients; the anatomical distribution having been recorded for 140 of these. *Table 2.8* illustrates the anatomical distribution of all recorded Grade 4 pressure ulcers. In Italy and Portugal at least 50% of all Grade 4 pressure ulcers were located at the sacrum while in Sweden and the United Kingdom most Grade 4 pressure ulcers were found over the heels.

Preventive care (defined as either the provision of a pressure redistributing support surface or regular manual repositioning) was recorded for all surveyed patients. Given the wide range of specialist mattresses and cushions in use across Europe, no attempt has been made during the EPUAP pilot pressure ulcer prevalence survey to identify individual products, rather all support surfaces are defined as being non-specialist (eg. standard mattress), non-powered (for example, low pressure foam mattresses) or powered (any device with a mains electrical supply). Regular repositioning was recorded as either not planned or allocated, or reported to be performed at differing time intervals. It should be noted that it was not possible to verify whether reported repositioning was in fact performed.

Table 2.8: Anatomical distribution of all Grade 4 pressure ulcers (n=140) shown by country. Data shows absolute numbers of pressure ulcers and the percentage, shown in parenthesis, within each category

Location	Belgium	Italy	Portugal	Sweden	United Kingdom	Total
Sacrum	7 (36.8)	12 (80.0)	12 (50.0)	4 (33.3)	22 (31.4)	57
Heels	5 (26.3)	2 (13.3)	5 (20.8)	6 (50.0)	37 (52.8)	55
Hips	0	0	2 (8.3)	2 (16.7)	2 (2.8)	6
Other	7 (36.8)	1 (6.7)	5 (20.8)	0	9 (12.8)	22
Total	**19**	**15**	**24**	**12**	**70**	**140**

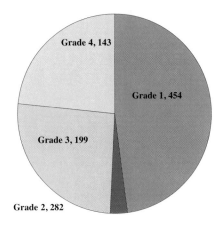

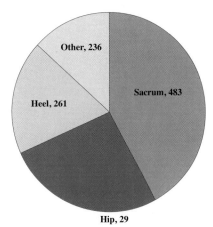

Figure 2.3: Severity of the most severe pressure ulcer experienced by the surveyed patients. The numbers adjacent to each slice of the chart give the absolute numbers of patients whose worst pressure ulcer was of this grade

Figure 2.4: Anatomical location of the most severe pressure ulcer experienced by the surveyed patients. The numbers adjacent to each slice of the chart give the absolute numbers of patients whose worst pressure ulcer was found at this body site. Location of the most severe pressure ulcer unreported in sixty-nine cases

To explore the allocation of preventive care, the surveyed patients have been divided into two groups; those considered vulnerable to pressure ulcer development (Braden score of 16 or below or with an established pressure ulcer regardless of its severity), and those patients considered to be at minimal risk of pressure damage (Braden score 17 or above and no pressure ulcers). This division provides an impression of the appropriateness of the allocation of preventive care and not an absolute measure, given the imperfect prediction of true vulnerability as provided by risk assessment tools such as the Braden scale.

Based upon these definitions or risk, 2114 (36.5%) patients were considered to be in need of preventive intervention. *Table 2.9* highlights the allocation of pressure-redistributing equipment while in bed and when seated for each country.

Table 2.9: The allocation of special beds, mattresses and cushions to patients encountered during the prevalence survey

The allocation of special beds

	No special equipment		Non-powered device		Powered device	
	at risk[a]	no risk	at risk	no risk[d]	at risk	no risk[b]
Belgium	152	528	84	12	6	-
UK	98	272	147	211	122	16
Sweden	115	344	107	54	5	1
Italy	185	754	24	9	38	3
Total	**601**	**2130**	**870**	**1454**	**643**	**94**

The allocation of special cushions

	No special equipment		Non-powered device		Powered device	
	at risk[c]	no risk	at risk	no risk	at risk[e]	no risk
Portugal	207	533	35	7	-	-
Belgium	284	453	78	45	5	1
UK	587	1192	410	266	34	16
Sweden	177	382	50	17	-	-
Italy	241	761	6	5	-	-
Total	**1496**	**3321**	**579**	**340**	**39**	**17**

Three columns have been highlighted in *Table 2.9* to focus attention upon areas where equipment allocation may be improved. Highlighted column (a) notes where patients assessed to be vulnerable to pressure damage were not allocated a pressure-redistributing mattress, whereas column (b) identifies instances where powered devices had been provided to patients apparently at minimal risk of developing pressure ulcers. Finally, column (c) notes where patients were at risk but not provided with a cushion; however, column (c) also included 871 bedfast patients that may have been expected not to have been allocated a cushion.

Interestingly, 138 bedfast patients were reported to have been allocated a special cushion! Of these, ninety-two were encountered in the United Kingdom (eight using powered cushions) with twenty-four in Portugal. Two further columns were identified in *Table 2.6*, column (d) marked an apparent high level of allocation of non-powered mattresses to patients at minimal risk, and this may mark hospitals where low-pressure foam mattresses were used as the standard bed mattress.

Finally, column (e) marks the general low provision of powered cushions regardless of patient vulnerability to pressure ulcer development.

Table 2.10 highlights the reported repositioning of patients by nursing staff. Most patients were not repositioned (for example, in bed, 4720 [81.6%] patients were not repositioned). Where patients at risk were not repositioned this may mark the allocation of special beds and mattresses. Interestingly, approximately 260 patients were re-positioned while in bed but did not appear to be vulnerable to pressure ulcer development.

A final indicator was developed from the data collected during the survey to mark the allocation of 'appropriate' preventive care. Appendix 4 to this chapter sets out the structure of the algorithm used to identify whether the recorded care was likely to be appropriate or potentially inappropriate. *Figure 2.5* identifies the proportion of patients who received appropriate or inappropriate preventive care. **While most patients in the participating countries received some preventive care, relatively few (*n*=265, 4.6%) were allocated fully appropriate care**. The percentage of the surveyed patients considered to receive adequate preventive care ranged from 0% (Italy) to 9.3% (United Kingdom).

Table 2.10: Reported repositioning of patients by nursing staff				
Reported repositioning of surveyed patients in bed by nursing staff				
	Yes		No	
	at risk	no risk	at risk	no risk
Portugal	39	9	203	531
Belgium	111	31	256	463
UK	454	163	577	1311
Sweden	76	11	151	388
Italy	127	46	120	720
Total	**807**	**260**	**1307**	**3413**
Reported repositioning of surveyed patients while seated by nursing staff				
	Yes		No	
	at risk	no risk	at risk	no risk
Portugal	5	4	237	536
Belgium	43	11	324	488
UK	271	148	760	1326
Sweden	26	12	201	387
Italy	44	43	203	723
Total	**389**	**218**	**1725**	**3460**

Conclusions

The European Pressure Ulcer Advisory Panel (EPUAP) has successfully undertaken a pilot study of the prevalence of pressure ulcers across a limited number of hospitals in five European countries. Overall, the prevalence of pressure ulcers was 18.1% (1078 of 5749 surveyed patients). Although differences were seen in the prevalence reported across different countries these cannot, by themselves, be used to mark differences in the quality or effectiveness of the care delivered. Clearly, the differences in prevalence proportion which ranged from 8.5% to 22.9% may have been influenced by differences in the patient population and their vulnerability to developing pressure ulcers. For these reasons, this report should not be used to compare and contrast the occurrence of pressure ulcers across the surveyed hospitals. Rather, the main value in this pilot study has been the large scale testing of a methodology through which the prevalence of pressure ulcers could be recorded; this methodology appears sufficiently robust for the EPUAP to recommend its adoption in future prevalence studies.

Across the 5947 surveyed patients, 143 (2.5%) were reported to experience the most severe form of pressure ulcer highlighting that effective prevention and treatment of pressure ulcers remains a high priority in acute care across Europe. This survey attempted to identify the appropriateness of the preventive care reported to be delivered; surprisingly, few patients apparently received fully appropriate interventions — with the percentage receiving such care ranging from 0% (Italy), to 0.5% (Portugal), 1.8% (Sweden), 2% (Belgium) with the highest percentage allocated appropriate preventive care found in the United Kingdom. However, even in the UK it was noted that fewer than 10% of the surveyed patients received fully adequate preventive care. These low percentages would suggest that there is much scope for the improvement of pressure ulcer preventive care across Europe.

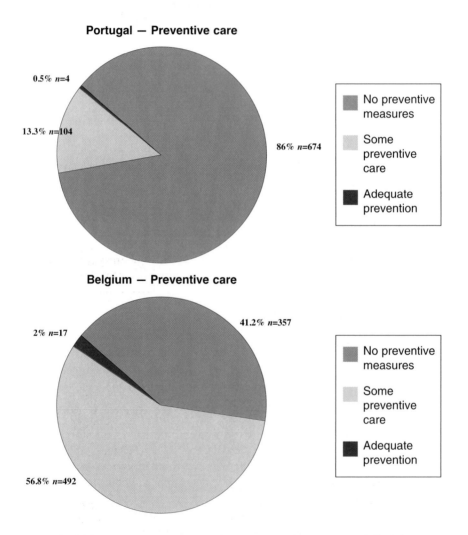

Figure 2.5: Assessment of preventive care allocated to the surveyed patients in the different countries

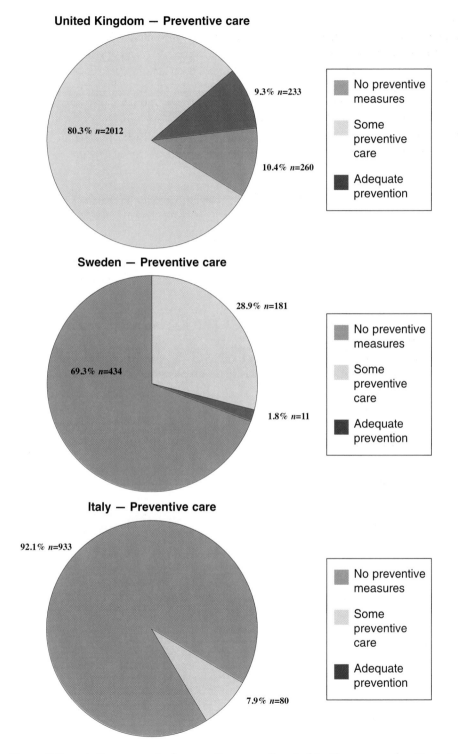

Figure 2.5 cont: Assessment of preventive care allocated to the surveyed patients in the different countries

> **Key points**
>
> ⌘ A methodology for collecting pressure ulcer prevalence data has been developed which can be used across national boundaries.
>
> ⌘ In a pilot study across twenty-six hospitals in five countries almost 20% of patients had a pressure ulcer. Relatively few patients received fully appropriate preventive care.
>
> ⌘ Despite considerable attention on pressure ulcers in recent years within Europe, there remains a long way to go before the challenge of pressure ulceration has been fully met.
>
> ⌘ Understanding reports of pressure ulcer occurrence rests upon the interpretation of the study methods. It is important that descriptions of the patient population and how pressure ulcers were reported are included in any report of prevalence or incidence.

Appendix 2.1: Members of the EPUAP Pressure Ulcer Prevalence Project Steering Group

Chair: Gerrie Bours, University of Maastricht, Department of Nursing Science, the Netherlands

Gerry Bennett, East London Wound Healing Centre, Royal London Hospital, United Kingdom

Michael Clark, Wound Healing Research Unit, University of Wales College of Medicine, United Kingdom

Carol Dealey is Research Fellow, Nursing and Therapy Research Unit, University of Birmingham and University Hospital Birmingham NHS Trust

Tom Defloor, University of Gent, Department of Nursing Science, Belgium

Jacqui Fletcher, University of Hertfordshire, United Kingdom

Ruud Halfens, University of Maastricht, Department of Nursing Science, the Netherlands

Sylvie Meaume, Groupe Hospitalier Charles Foix-jean Rostand, France

Appendix 2.2: EPUAP pressure ulcer prevalence data collection instrument

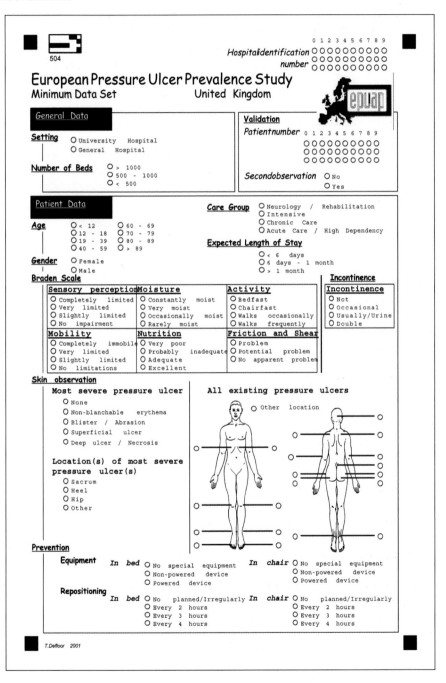

504

Hospital identification number
0 1 2 3 4 5 6 7 8 9

European Pressure Ulcer Prevalence Study
Minimum Data Set United Kingdom

General Data

Setting
O University Hospital
O General Hospital

Number of Beds
O > 1000
O 500 - 1000
O < 500

Validation

Patient number 0 1 2 3 4 5 6 7 8 9

Second observation
O No
O Yes

Patient Data

Age
O < 12   O 60 - 69
O 12 - 18   O 70 - 79
O 19 - 39   O 80 - 89
O 40 - 59   O > 89

Gender
O Female
O Male

Care Group
O Neurology / Rehabilitation
O Intensive
O Chronic Care
O Acute Care / High Dependency

Expected Length of Stay
O < 6 days
O 6 days - 1 month
O > 1 month

Braden Scale

Sensory perception	Moisture	Activity	Incontinence
O Completely limited	O Constantly moist	O Bedfast	**Incontinence**
O Very limited	O Very moist	O Chairfast	O Not
O Slightly limited	O Occasionally moist	O Walks occasionally	O Occasional
O No impairment	O Rarely moist	O Walks frequently	O Usually/Urine
			O Double

Mobility	Nutrition	Friction and Shear
O Completely immobile	O Very poor	O Problem
O Very limited	O Probably inadequate	O Potential problem
O Slightly limited	O Adequate	O No apparent problem
O No limitations	O Excellent	

Skin observation

Most severe pressure ulcer
O None
O Non-blanchable erythema
O Blister / Abrasion
O Superficial ulcer
O Deep ulcer / Necrosis

Location(s) of most severe pressure ulcer(s)
O Sacrum
O Heel
O Hip
O Other

All existing pressure ulcers
O Other location

Prevention

Equipment
In bed
O No special equipment
O Non-powered device
O Powered device

In chair
O No special equipment
O Non-powered device
O Powered device

Repositioning
In bed
O No planned/Irregularly
O Every 2 hours
O Every 3 hours
O Every 4 hours

In chair
O No planned/Irregularly
O Every 2 hours
O Every 3 hours
O Every 4 hours

T.Defloor 2001

Appendix 2.3: The EPUAP pressure ulcer classification system

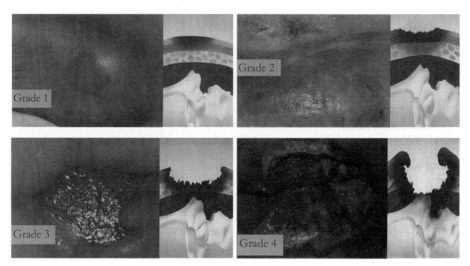

Line diagrams reproduced by kind permission of Huntleigh Healthcare Limited

Appendix 2.4: Elements of the care allocated to patients considered to mark fully appropriate pressure ulcer preventive care

A patient was deemed to receive fully appropriate preventive care if they were allocated one of the following combinations:

- ⌘ powered device in bed and powered device in chair
- ⌘ powered device in bed and non-powered device in chair and repositioning in chair every two or three hours
- ⌘ powered device in bed and bedfast (activity Braden scale)
- ⌘ non-powered device in bed and repositioning in bed every two, three or four hours and powered device in chair
- ⌘ non-powered device in bed and repositioning in bed every two, three or four hours and non-powered device in chair and repositioning in chair every two or three hours
- ⌘ non-powered device in bed and repositioning in bed every two, three or four hours and bedfast (activity Braden scale)
- ⌘ no device in bed and repositioning in bed every two hours and powered device in chair
- ⌘ no device in bed and repositioning in bed every two hours and non-powered device in chair and repositioning in chair every two or three hours
- ⌘ no device in bed and repositioning in bed every two hours and bedfast.

3

Case-mix adjusted incidence of pressure ulcers in acute medical and surgical wards

Susan Williams, Lynne Watret, and Jill Pell

Pressure ulcers cause considerable pain and suffering and are also a very expensive drain on NHS funding. Measuring prevalence is particularly useful for guiding use of resources, whereas incidence is an outcome indicator of quality of care. Patients and illnesses vary and it may be misleading to make assumptions based on crude incidence figures. A system of case-mix adjustment has been developed in Glasgow (GPSISS). This study used GPSISS to measure case-mix adjusted incidence of pressure ulcers in over 15 000 acute hospital patients. The incidence of pressure ulcers ranged from 1.1% to 2.7%. These low rates, and the time, cost and effort involved in ensuring quality data, suggests that significant differences in quality of care may be demonstrated more quickly using processes rather than outcomes, and may more directly identify where changes in practice are required.

Background

Measuring point prevalence (*Box 3.1*) is an effcient method of assessing need for resources for patients who have established pressure ulcers and its advantages and disadvantages have been widely reported (O'Dea, 1993, 1995; St Clair *et al*, 1995; Pieper *et al*, 1998). In Glasgow, we were interested in the quality of preventative pressure ulcer care delivered to adults admitted to acute hospitals. Measuring crude incidence (*Box 3.1*) is limited since it makes no allowance for any variation in health status (Clark, 1998; Berlowitz *et al*, 1996; James *et al*, 1998). We developed a method of taking into account variations between patients and the effects of their illnesses – the Glasgow Pressure Sore Incidence Scoring System (GPSISS). The method was successfully piloted in two Glasgow hospitals (Williams *et al*, 1997).

Case-mix adjustment (*Box 3.1*) allows for comparing 'like with like' and GPSISS is based on two practical factors which reflect health status and are easily recorded – length of hospital stay and the Waterlow Pressure Ulcer Risk Assessment Score (Waterlow, 1985). Patients are classified into sixteen sub-groups of risk based on permutations of their highest Waterlow score (0–9, 10–14, 15–19 and 20+) and length of stay (0–7, 8–14, 15–21 and 22+ days). Case-mix adjusted incidence of pressure ulcers in each unit is then calculated using indirect standardisation. This compares the 'observed' number of ulcers that actually occurred in a unit with the 'expected' number. This is the number estimated to have occurred had each unit had the same patient characteristics as the standard population (all unit populations combined) (Williams *et al*, 1997).

This chapter describes the results of a study to measure the case-mix adjusted incidence of pressure ulcers, using GPSISS, in adults admitted to all acute adult medical and surgical wards of Glasgow NHS hospitals.

⌘ **Pressure ulcer** — a new break in the skin or worse over a pressure point, following admission to hospital

⌘ **Point prevalence of pressure ulcers** — the total number of people in a defined population with pressure ulcers at a specified time

⌘ **Crude incidence** — the number of people developing a new pressure ulcer involving a break in the skin or worse who are admitted to a designated unit, eg. ward, directorate or hospital, over a set period of time

⌘ **Case-mix adjusted incidence** — crude incidence adjusted for varying health status judged in terms of the Waterlow Risk Assessment Score and length of hospital stay

⌘ **Confidence intervals** — allows for a level of uncertainty of actual value — range of values that confidently includes the true value (Altman D [1991] *Practical Statistics for Medical Research*. Chapman and Hall, London)

⌘ **Inter-rater reliability** — the level of agreement between individuals when using the same measuring tool

Box 3.1: Definitions of terms used in the text

Sample and methods

To provide meaningful statistical interpretation of data, a minimum of 1350 medical and 1350 surgical patients from each hospital were required for the study. The rationale for these sample sizes was based on a case-mix adjusted difference in incidence of 3.4% between the two hospitals in the pilot study. Power calculations indicated that in order to demonstrate if a difference of this magnitude would be statistically significant at the 5% level, data would be required on 1332 patients (Williams *et al*, 1997). From the pilot study we knew it was possible to achieve almost complete collection of data, however, to allow for attrition sample sizes of 1350 were targeted.

Patients were eligible for the study if they were admitted to either acute medical or surgical wards over two six-month periods in 1996 and 1997. They were then followed up for a maximum period of twenty-eight days or until death or discharge if this occurred first. Skin assessment, using the Waterlow Risk Assessment Score (Waterlow, 1985) was undertaken daily by qualified ward nurses. Information was then recorded on forms specially designed for the study. A separate form was completed for each patient and followed the patient throughout their stay in hospital.

The Waterlow Risk Assessment Score is used in Glasgow because it is well established and is based on a variety of risk factors including height-weight ratio, skin type, sex, age, continence, mobility, appetite and specific diseases and drugs (Waterlow, 1985). Identification of specific risk factors provides an important opportunity for care to be tailored to individual need.

In Glasgow, it is policy, that on admission to any ward patients are risk assessed for pressure ulcers and this should be repeated if there is a change in the patient's condition or circumstances. Confidence in nurses' ability to risk assess accurately was based on earlier local audits which indicated that by the end of 1995, 769 hours had been dedicated to teaching nurses of all grades, including over 1592 trained nurses, how to use the Waterlow Risk Assessment Score and the Torrance Grading System (Waterlow, 1985; Torrance, 1983). Teaching included practice at scoring based on case scenarios and grading using slide presentations. Local audits and spot checks by the tissue viability nurses confirmed that whilst nurses were not always accurate at using the Torrance Grading System, they were skilled at risk assessing using Waterlow.

The Torrance Grading System (Torrance, 1983) is in established use in Glasgow because it is quick and straightforward to implement. In order to remove ambiguity, in light of the knowledge that grading was not always accurate, especially in relation to grade 1 and 2 ulcers, nurses also recorded whether or not any new break in the skin was present. This was accepted as the definition of a pressure ulcer for the purpose of the study (*Box 3.1*).

The study was supervised by a half-time F-grade nurse at each of the five hospitals. Their duties included; visiting the wards daily to ensure that all new patients had been recruited to the study, undertaking inter-rater reliability checks (*Box 3.1*) on Waterlow scoring, training nurses in the measurement of incidence, supervising data collection and quality of recordings, assessing the completeness of recruitment by checking admission lists, and collating and coding of data. The cost of employing these data managers over the two six-month periods was £48 000.

Data for the medical and surgical wards were analysed separately and then combined, using SPSS and Excel. The case-mix adjusted incidence of pressure ulcers was calculated for each hospital separately and compared with the incidence calculated for all five hospitals combined (Williams *et al*, 1997).

Results

Data were collected on 15 346 (7417 medical and 7929 surgical) patients. Data were complete for over 99% of admissions. This level of completeness can be credited to the employment of dedicated data mangers at each site and their thoroughness at supervising and checking comprehensiveness of data.

Varying patient characteristics

Overall, during their hospital stay, 9019 (59%) patients remained at a low risk of developing pressure ulcers according to their Waterlow score (<10) and 2698 (17%) were classified as high risk or very high risk (≥15). Six hundred and fourteen (4%) were reclassified into high or very high-risk categories during their hospital stay. Similarly, medium risk classifications rose by 1% and consequently low risk classifications fell by 5% (*Figure 3.1*). There was a statistically significant difference between the hospitals in the breakdown of patients by highest Waterlow score (χ^2 test=50.4, d/f=12, *P*=<0.001) and lengths of stay of patients (χ^2 test=122.5, d/f=12, *P*=<0.001). Overall, 14 112 (92%) were discharged within two weeks and over three quarters were discharged within one week of admission. As would be expected, medical patients stayed in hospital for longer and 11% were still in hospital after two weeks compared with 6% of surgical patients (χ^2 test=124, d/f=1, *P*=<0.001).

Incidence of pressure ulcers

Two hundred and seventy-one (150 medical and 121 surgical) patients developed a new break in the skin giving an overall crude incidence of 2%. However this varied from 0.8% in surgical patients to 2.6% in medical patients in Hospital 2, a difference of 1.8% (*Table 3.1*). When medical and surgical wards were scrutinised separately and adjustments were made for case-mix in terms of highest Waterlow score and length of hospital stay, differences were observed which reinforced the importance of case-mix

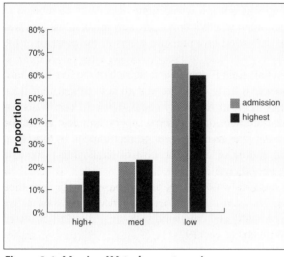

Figure 3.1: Varying Waterlow categories

adjustment in providing fair comparisons (*Table 3.1*). Case-mix adjustment had most impact on the Hospital 2 surgical patients, where crude incidence was the lowest (0.8%) but with case-mix adjustment became the highest (2.2%) a difference of 1.4%. Thus, based on crude incidence rates, the surgical wards in Hospital 2 appeared to be most successful at preventing pressure damage and therefore may be expected to have delivered high quality preventive care. However, the increased case-mix adjusted rate suggested that these patients had better health status compared to those at the other hospitals and therefore worse outcomes when this was taken into account. The converse was true for Hospital 5 medical patients (*Table 3.1*), where a high crude incidence rate of 2.5% was adjusted to 1.1% due to the apparent poorer health status of their patients.

Table 3.1: Crude and case-mix adjusted incidence of pressure ulcers in medical and surgical wards

	Hospital 1	Hospital 2	Hospital 3	Hospital 4	Hospital 5	Overall
Medical wards						
Crude incidence	1.3%	2.6%	2.3%	1.4%	2.5%	2.0%
Case-mix adjusted incidence	1.1%	2.7%	2.5%	2.5%	1.1%	
(95% CI)	(0.6 to 1.6%)	(1.9 to 3.5%)	(1.6 to 3.4%)	(1.4 to 3.3%)	(0.5 to 1.5%)	(1.9 to 2.1%)
Surgical wards						
Crude incidence	1.5%	0.8%	1.1%	2.2%	2.1%	2.0%
Case-mix adjusted incidence	1.4%	2.2%	1.1%	2.1%	2%	
(95% CI)	(0.9 to 2.1%)	(1.5 to 3%)	(0.6 to 1.6%)	(1.4 to 3%)	(1.3 to 2.7%)	(1.1 to 2.5%)

Confidence intervals (*Box 3.1*) also indicated that the case-mix adjusted rates in medical patients in Hospitals 1 and 5 were significantly lower than that of all medical patients (*Table 3.1*) (ie. the highest levels for Hospital 1 of 1.6% and for Hospital 5 of 1.5% were lower than the lower confidence level of 1.9% overall). This indicates that in terms of pressure ulcer prevention in medical wards, Hospitals 1 and 5 are significantly better than the Glasgow hospitals overall.

Severity of ulcers

Two hundred and fifty-five (1.6%) patients developed a grade 2 or 3 ulcer whilst in hospital. Sixteen (<1%) (9 medical and 7 surgical) developed a grade 4 or 5 ulcer.

Conclusions

The study successfully measured case-mix adjusted incidence of pressure ulcers. High quality data were collected on over 15,000 patients and case-mix adjustment allowed for more meaningful comparisons between hospitals.

Incidence was low in both medical and surgical wards. This was of interest because our pilot study, to test the methodology, had found case-mix adjusted rates of rates of 6.3% and 9.7% (Williams *et al*, 1997). This difference might indicate a genuine improvement in care. However, it may be due to the inclusion in the pilot figures of patients with pre-existing ulcers or skin which was red but not broken. This seems the more likely reason for the difference because of the similarities between the hospitals in the case-mix adjusted incidence rates recorded in the main study, whether or not the hospital had taken part in the pilot study. For the main study, we had taken the precaution of reinforcing on the data collection sheets completed by the clinical nurses the information that only new breaks in the skin should be recorded. The data managers were also primed to check that all the correct information was being recorded. Based on these reinforcements, together with the completeness of recruitment, we are confident that the data collected in the main study were robust. The low rates recorded in the study should be considered a minimum measure of incidence because of the short time spent in hospital by most patients. It is possible that ulcers sustained as a result of hospital stay might not be evident until after discharge and therefore not recorded. In the pilot-study, attempts to follow-up all high-risk patients at home by telephone had to be abandoned. Over half were not immediately contactable and follow-up proved to be time-consuming and expensive. Many were not referred to the community nursing service.

The longer the stay in hospital, the greater the likelihood of developing damage. It would be a reasonable assumption that such patients are in hospital longer because of their poorer health status and therefore more dependent. The majority of pressure ulcers which were recorded as part of this study were superficial, no matter the length of a patient's stay. This reflects Pieper *et al*'s (1998) observation that nosocomial pressure ulcers tend to be of a lower grade than ulcers present on admission. It was also noted that pressure damage was more likely to occur when the Waterlow Risk Assessment Score was at its highest, thus validating score predictability and suggesting an acute change in the patient's condition or an overall deterioration in their health predisposes to a pressure ulcer. This highlighted the need for regular patient assessment with corresponding review of their care plan to ensure quality of care.

Measuring the incidence of pressure ulcers effectively takes time, is labour intensive and relatively expensive to supervise properly. The low rates in this study may reflect high standards of care or, as indicated, may be because most patients do not remain in hospital long enough for an ulcer to develop. Whatever the reason, the low rates indicate that using incidence to measure quality of care in acute settings is not an effcient use of resources. Also, this outcome measure is limited in that it does not identify the deficiencies in care which may lead to pressure ulcers. Additional information about actual nursing management collected with the incidence data for the surgical patients proved more useful in identifying quickly where improvements needed to be made. We therefore recommend that quality of care in relation to pressure ulcers is most effciently assessed using process rather than outcome measures.

Finally, the complete picture is important and it would be valuable to have some information on the number and type of pressure ulcers developing in patients recently discharged from acute hospital care. We recommend that closer liaison between nurses working in acute care and their colleagues working in the community, including nursing homes, should take place and that post discharge pressure ulcers should be treated as critical incidents. A study to test the feasibility of this approach is planned.

Key points

⌘ Comparing pressure ulcer prevalence or incidence rates can be misleading if no account is taken of potential differences between the surveyed populations, for example, changes in age, vulnerability to pressure ulcers and general medical condition.

⌘ This chapter has presented one approach to developing comparable pressure ulcer occurence data. It is now time for all reports of pressure ulcer occurrence to present data adjusted to reflect the characteristics of the surveyed population.

⌘ Risk adjustment is not 'rocket science' but it is essential if true comparisons in clinical centres and over time are to be made.

References

Berlowitz D, Ash A, Brandeis G, Harriet K, Halpern J, Moskowitz A (1996) Rating long term care facilities on pressure ulcer development: importance of case-mix adjustment. *Ann Intern Med* **124**(6): 557–63

Clark M (1998) Removing the 'estimates and guesses' from practice – evidence based tissue viability. *J Tissue Viability* **8**(2): 3–5

James G, Nicholl J, Slack R, Pirie P, McClemont E (1998) *Setting targets: achieving reductions in pressure sores.* University of Sheffield, Sheffield

O'Dea K (1993) The prevalence of pressure damage in UK hospitals. *J Wound Care* **2**(4): 221–5

O'Dea K (1995) The prevalence of pressure ulcers in four European countries. *J Wound Care* **4**(4): 192–5

Pieper B, Sugrue M, Weiland M, Sprague K, Heiman C (1998) Risk factors, prevention methods and wound care for patients with pressure ulcers. *Clinical Nurse Specialist* **12**(1): 7–12

St Clair M, Cooper S, Gebhardt K (1995) Measuring pressure sore incidence: a study. *Nurs Standard* **9**(19): 50–1

Torrance C (1983) *Pressure Sore Aetiology, Treatment and Prevention.* Croom Helm, Beckenham

Williams S, Jackson B, Watret L, Pell J (1997) Pilot study of case-mix adjusted incidence of pressure sores. *J Tissue Viability* **7**(1): 15–19

Waterlow J (1985) Waterlow: a risk assessment card. *Nurs Times* **81**(48): 49–51

Section II:
Risk factors: facts and fallacies

We cannot hope to build the use of effective interventions into our pressure ulcer prevention and treatment practices if we do not understand the complex aetiology of pressure ulcers — for how can we effectively prevent or treat when the specific causes are unclear? Many read, and accept, simplistic models of pressure ulcer formation which tend to imply that high pressures (and in the minds of many high means over 32mmHg) cut off the blood supply to the tissues, which then die and a pressure ulcer is born! If such models were the entire story, then the widespread use of pressure-redistributing support surfaces seen since the mid 1980s would have eradicated the problem of pressure ulcers — this has not occurred. The simplistic story does not take account of many extrinsic and intrinsic factors that can accelerate or ameliorate the effects of prolonged compression — if we are to fully understand pressure ulcers we need to determine the complex interactions between these myriad factors. This section explores aspects of the basic anatomical structure of tissues liable to pressure ulceration; such fundamental work is required but has too often been overlooked in the rush to compare the effects of different interventions on pressure ulcer prevention and treatment. The section also serves to illustrate the interest in pressure ulcers that currently exists in Japan — there is a clear need for the several groups of pressure ulcer workers worldwide to be aware of each organisation's activity and to seek common areas for joint projects. The second chapter in this section provides a scholarly review of the biological significance and measurement of interface pressures — this measure has been subject to misunderstanding and misrepresentation within acres of manufacturers' supporting literature until many practitioners have little insight into the true value potential of interface pressure measurements. This chapter cuts through the confusion and helps to reclaim interface pressure measurement as one tool available to understand pressure ulceration.

4

Morphological architecture and distribution of blood capillaries and elastic fibres in the human skin

Satsue Hagisawa, Tatsuo Shimada, Hiromi Arao and Yuji Asada

This study was undertaken to clarify the morphological features in the blood capillary and elastic fibre distribution of the human skin in terms of susceptibility to pressure ulcer development. Skin tissues were obtained from bony areas: the sacrum and ischial tuberosity, and non-bony area: the centre of the gluteus maximus of five aged subjects post mortem for examination using light and scanning electron microscopy. It was observed that the sacral skin had finger-like papillae and underneath the blood capillary loops were most numerous. In the ischial skin, the dermal papillae consisted of a combination of finger-like and trapezoid shapes having moderate density of blood capillaries. In contrast, the dermal papillae in the gluteal skin were almost flat, so that the blood capillaries were scattered. The size of elastic bundles in the papillary layer of the sacral, ischial and gluteal skin ranged from 2 to 3 μm, 5 to 10 μm, and 3 to 5 μm, respectively. The elastic fibres were densely distributed in the ischial skin while less so in the sacral skin.

Introduction

It is generally accepted that pressure sores result from prolonged and/or repeated ischaemic insults without adequate time for total tissue recovery resulting in tissue necrosis, although the cause of the condition is multifactorial. The external pressure over bony prominences will decrease the skin blood flow causing lack of oxygen and nutrients in the tissues. The most susceptible areas of the body to pressure insults are the sacrum in the supine and the ischial tuberosities in the sitting positions, both of which are bony prominences experiencing localized pressure when the body position is not changed. On the other hand, the site over the centre of the gluteus maximus is a non-bony area having a lot of subcutaneous tissues acting as a 'cushion' to distribute the force applied.

It is assumed that tissue viability depends on blood capillary density, vascular response to pressure and underlying tissue recovery behavior after pressure release. The vascular response to pressure has been examined in many studies as a postischaemic reactive hyperemia in association with susceptibility of pressure sore development (Schubert and Fagrell, 1991; Hagisawa *et al*, 1994; Kabagambe *et al*, 1994). However, little is known about blood capillary and elastic fibre distribution in the skin, both of which may also significantly affect the tissue viability of the skin following ischaemia. The blood capillaries located under the dermal papillae provide the oxygen and nutrition to the tissues. Pasyk *et al* (1989) reported regional differences in blood capillary density of the human papillary dermis biopsied at twenty different areas from six cadavers, ranging in age from sixty to eighty years. They concluded that higher capillary density was observed in the head-face/neck region than in the lower parts of the body. The elastic fibres, which are situated in the papillary and reticular layers, play an important role in facilitating tissue recovery from the deformation following loading. There is a report examining elastic fibrils of the skin in patients with amyotrophic lateral sclerosis (Provinciali *et al*, 1994); however, the skin sample examined was obtained from the forearm which may have different features to bony areas such as the sacrum and ischium. If blood capillary and elastic fibres are not densely distributed in a loaded area, tissue recovery from ischaemia will be delayed leading to increasing tissue insult.

This study was undertaken to clarify the morphological features and distribution of both blood capillaries and elastic fibres in the skin of bony areas, including the sacrum and the ischial tuberosity. The distribution over bony prominences was then compared with a non-bony area, the centre of the gluteus maximus.

Materials and methods

Human skin tissues without pressure sores were excised from five aged subjects post mortem, six to eight hours after death. Detailed information about these subjects such as age, sex, cause of death and mobility before death is provided in *Table 4.1*. The skin tissues were obtained from three different sites of the body: sacrum, ischial tuberosity and over the centre of gluteus maximus (*Figure 4.1*).

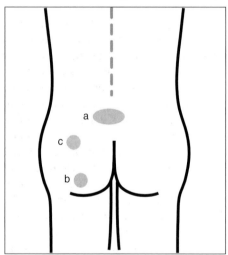

Figure 4.1: Sites of the body where the skin tissues were obtained: a. sacrum; b, ischial tuberosity; c. centre of gluteus maximus

The skin samples were processed for examination by light microscopy (LM) and scanning electron microscopy (SEM).

1. Light microscopy

For the observation of blood capillary in the papillary layer, the skin tissues were fixed in 4% paraformaldehyde in 0.1 M cacodylate buffer, pH 7.4, for two to three hours. Frozen sections, 30 μm in thickness, were cut with a cryostat, mounted on albumin-coated glass slides and air-dried. For alkaline phosphatase (ALPase) reaction, they were incubated for 60–120 minutes at 4°C using the azo-dye method, coverslipped with glycerin jelly and photographed using a light microscope (Nikon-Optiphot, Japan).

A small block of skin tissues was also fixed in 10% formalin and embedded in paraffin and thick sections (i5 μm) were stained with resorcin-fuchsin and kernechtrot to emphasize the demonstration of elastic fibres.

2. Scanning electron microscopy

Skin tissues with about 1 cm square were fixed in a mixture of 2.5% glutaraldehyde and 2% paraformaldehyde in 0.1 M cacodylate buffer, pH 7.4, for two hours or longer at

4°C. In order to digest collagen fibres of the dermis, the tissues were treated with 6N NaOH for ten to fifteen minutes at 60°C. Then they were rinsed thoroughly in distilled water (DW), immersed in 1% tannic acid/DW for two hours, placed in 1% OsO_4/DW for two hours, dehydrated in a graded series of

Table 4.1: Subjects

Subject no	Age	Sex	Cause of death	Mobility before death
1	92	M	Lung cancer	2 days bedridden
2	75	M	Liver cancer	Good mobility
3	73	F	Lung cancer	Unknown
4	67	F	Gastric cancer	Unknown
5	83	F	Acute renal failure	Unknown

ethanol and dried by the *t*-butylalcohol freeze drying method. The specimens were coated with gold and viewed using a scanning electron microscope (Hitachi S-800, Japan).

Results

It was found that the tendency of the morphological features observed at the sacral, ischial and gluteal skin was similar among all five subjects.

1. Light microscopic findings

In the frozen sections reacted for ALPase, arterioles, capillaries were stained a dark blue but venules were not stained. Blood capillaries were widely distributed in the papillary layer and their microvascular architectures showed considerable differences depending on the sites of the skin. The finger-like papillae seemed to have a lot of blood capillaries underneath while flat or trapezoid papillae did not. The loops of blood capillaries found in the dermal papillary ridges were most numerous in the sacral skin (*Figure 4.2a*). In the ischial skin the dermal papillae consisted of two types of configuration: finger-like papillae possessing the capillary loops and large trapezoid papillae having loose capillary nets (*Figure 4.2b*). In contrast, the gluteal skin had no dermal papillae and blood capillaries appeared to be scattered (*Figure 4.2c*). In paraffin sections of skin tissues stained with resorcinfuchsin and kernechtrot, elastic fibres were stained a violet color and were distributed abundantly between bundles of collagen fibres in the reticular layers of the all dermis obtained (*Figures 4.3a–c*). The reticular layer of the dermis consisted of dense and irregular connective tissues, in which collagen fibres were relatively coarse and interwoven in a compact meshwork. Elastic fibres were usually interspersed among the collagen fibres. Elastic fibres in the reticular layers of the sacral skin were interspersed compared with ischial and gluteal skin.

Fine elastic fibres were detected in the papillary layer of the dermis. It was noted that not only the configuration of the dermal papillae but also the distribution of elastic fibres in the papillary layer varied considerably among the three different sites on the skin.

It was found that in the sacral skin, which had numerous dermal papillae, the elastic fibres were relatively less dense compared with the ischial and gluteal skin (*Figure 4.3a*). The ischial skin had finger-like and trapezoid dermal papillae and the numerous elastic fibres in the papillary layer were more widely distributed compared with other two sites (*Figure 4.3b*). In the gluteal skin the dermal papillae was almost flat, although the density of elastic fibres was moderate in sacral and ischial skin (*Figure 4.3c*).

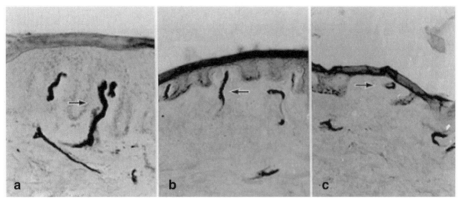

Figure 4.2: Light micrographs showing blood capillaries (arrows) underneath the human dermal papillae (x 140). Tissue sections were stained by the ALPase reaction. The blood capillary loops were most numerous in the sacral skin: a. sacral skin; b. ischial skin; c. gluteal skin

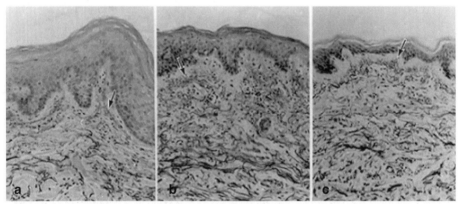

Figure 4.3: Light micrographs showing elastic fibre distribution in the human papillary layers (x 210). Tissue sections were stained with resoucin-fuchsin. A high density of elastic fibres (arrows) was observed in the ischial skin: a. sacral skin; b. ischial skin; c. gluteal skin

2. Scanning electron microscopic findings

When the human skin tissues were immersed in 6N NaOH solution at 60°C for ten minutes, the epidermis was successfully removed and the dermis was exposed. From SEM observations, it was confirmed that the configuration of the dermal papillae was similar to that observed in light microscopy, namely, the papillae in the sacral, ischial and gluteal skin showed a finger-like, mixed configuration of finger-like and trapezoid, respectively. Most of the superficial surface of the dermis was covered with dense networks of reticulin fibrils, which were about 40 μm in diameter (*Figure 4.4*).

Furthermore, the treatment of the skin tissues with 6N NaOH solution at 60°C for fifteen minutes enabled the observation of elastic fibres and free nerve endings in the papillary layer three-dimensionally. Elastic fibres consisted of bundles of fine elastic fibrils and were freely distributed within a loose network. SEM observation established definitely that the size and density of elastic fibres differed in different sites on the skin

(*Figure 4.5a–c*). The size of elastic bundles in the papillary layer of the sacral, ischial and gluteal skin ranged from 2 to 3 µm, 5 to 10 µm and 3 to 5 µm, respectively. A high density of elastic fibres was observed in the ischial skin (*Figure 4.5b*) while low density in the sacral skin (*Figure 4.5a*) and moderate in the gluteal skin (*Figure 4.5c*). In addition, free nerve endings were characterized by the presence of bead-like varicosities and reticular nets. A high density of them was observed in the sacral skin (*Figure 4.5a*) with a low density in the gluteal skin (*Figure 4.5c*).

These findings are summarized in *Table 4.2*.

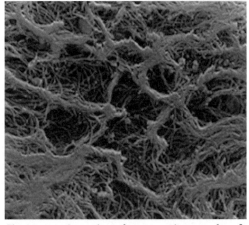

Figure 4.4: Scanning electron micrographs of dense networks of reticulin fibrils covering the most superficial surface of the dermis (x 9000)

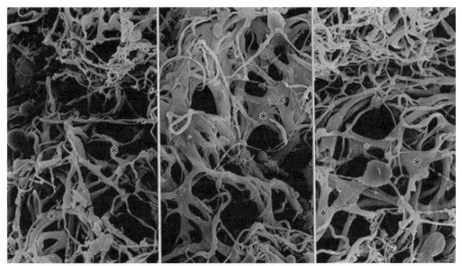

Figure 4.5: Scanning electron micrographs showing elastic bundle distribution in the human papillary layers (x 1300). The skin tissues were treated with NaOH to digest reticulin and collagen fibres. Thick elastic bundles (asterisks) were densely distributed in the ischial skin: a. sacral skin; b. ischial skin; c. gluteal skin

Table 4.2: Summary of the results obtained

Site	Shape of dermal papillae	Capillary density	Size of elastic bundle	Elastic bundle density
Sacrum	Finger-like	High	2-3 µm	Low
Ischial tuberosity	Finger-like + trapezoid	Moderate	5–10 µm	Highest
Centre of gluteus maximus	Almost flat (trapezoid)	Low	3–5 µm	Higher

Discussion

1. Sacral skin

It is recognized that the sacral area is prone to the development of pressure sores because of a bony prominence where compressive forces are concentrated when a person lies down. It was observed that the density of blood capillaries in the sacral skin was higher compared to the other two sites, and less of elastic fibres. It is likely that the sacral region in the elderly becomes more bony with aging and has had experience of loading frequently when lying. The force-related stimulation may facilitate development of the papillae in the upper dermis, as seen in the fingers which are always exposed to various forces. Dense distribution of blood capillaries is a good prognostic indicator for maintenance of tissue viability following ischaemia. However, the density of elastic fibres was less compared with other sites. This may suggest that tissue recovery from deformation produced by loading may be delayed. This might be one of the reasons why the sacrum is susceptible to pressure sore formation in spite of dense blood capillary distribution.

2. Ischial skin

The ischial tuberosities are known weight-bearing sites. Most of the body weight is concentrated in that area to support the upper trunk when a person is seated. The interface pressure at the ischial tuberosity is around 150–200 mmHg (Lindan and Greenway, 1965; Houle, 1969), which is likely to be higher than capillary pressure (Landis, 1930), depending on the hardness of support surface and underlying soft tissues. In this study it was observed that the blood capillary distribution in the ischial skin was between that of sacral and gluteal skin, while the thick elastic fibres were distributed densely compared with the other two sites. It is assumed that the elastic fibres observed at this site enable the buttock muscles to stretch or contract for any leg movements including sitting and standing. It is suggested that the thick elastic fibres densely distributed in the ischial skin may greatly contribute to tissue recovery from deformation, which may facilitate the blood capillaries to recover from ischaemia too. The frequent body movements resulting from normal activity also facilitate this phenomenon. Therefore, the skin over the ischial tuberosity is likely to be resistant to pressure despite frequent loading during daily activities.

3. Gluteal skin

In contrast to the sacral skin, it was found that there were very few blood capillaries in the gluteal skin, although the elastic fibres were moderately distributed. The scattered blood capillary distribution seen in this non-bony area may indicate that the nutrient requirement of the skin is low. If a site with fewer blood capillaries and elastic fibres is compressed for a prolonged period of time, although it is unlikely, tissue tolerance to pressure might be less.

It should be noted, however, that the main limitation in this study is that the skin samples obtained were all from aged subjects. It is known that the blood capillary and elastic fibre distribution is different in aged subjects compared with younger ones (Rickey *et al*, 1988) and between different sites even in the same subject (Pasyk *et al*, 1989). Further study is needed to determine how the distribution of blood capillaries and elastic fibres with collagen fibres in the skin differs at various sites on the body and among different age groups, in particular in susceptible areas to pressure sore formation.

Conclusion

Sacral skin was characterized by a dense distribution of blood capillaries, but less elastic fibres in the dermal papillae. In the gluteal skin, blood capillaries were scattered, but a moderate distribution of elastic fibres was observed. Ischial skin had moderate density of blood capillaries and densely distributed thick elastic fibres.

Key points

⌘ It is unlikely that significant advances in pressure ulcer prevention will be achieved in the absence of detailed understanding of a physical structure of the skin and soft tissues at vulnerable anatomical sites.

⌘ Basic pathology of the areas liable to pressure ulcers has been largely overlooked in recent years with the assumption that enough is known about the causes of pressure ulcers! Such views are incorrect, for knowledge of the mechanisms of pressure damage remain relatively illusive.

⌘ This chapter presents data illustrating morphological differences between areas prone to pressure ulcers and other parts of the human body, and illustrates one current focus of the highly active pressure ulcer research conducted in Japan.

References

Schubert V, Fagrell B (1991) Evaluation of the dynamic cutaneous postischaemic hyperaemia and thermal response in elderly subjects and in an area at risk for pressure sores. *Clinical Physiology* **11**: 169–82

Hagisawa S, Ferguson-Pell M, Cardi M, Miller SD (1994) Assessment of skin blood content and oxygenation in spinal cord injured subjects during reactive hyperemia. *J Rehabil Res Dev* **31**: 1–14

Kabagambe MK, Swain I, Shakespeare P (1994) An investigation of the effects of local pressure on the microcirculation of the skin (reactive hyperemia) in spinal cord injured patients. *J Tissue Viability* **4**(4): 110–23

Pasyk KA, Thomas SV, Hassett CA, Cherry GW, Faller R (1989) Regional differences in capillary density of the normal human dermis. *Plast Reconstr Surg* **83**(6): 939–47

Provinciali L, Cangiotti A, Tulli D, Carboni V, Cinti S (1994) Skin abnormalities involvement in the early stage of amyotrophic lateral sclerosis. *J Neurol Sci* **126**: 54–61

Lindan O, Greenway RM (1965) Pressure distribution on the surface of the human body: 1. Evaluation in lying and sitting positions using a 'bed of springs and nails'. *Arch Phys Med Rehabil* **46**: 378–85

Houle RJ (1969) Evaluation of seat devices designed to prevent ischemic ulcers in paraplegic patients. *Arch Phys Med Rehabil* **50**: 587–94

Landis EM (1930) Micro-injection studies of capillary blood pressure in human skin. *Heart* **15**: 209–28

Rickey ML, Rickey HK, Fenske NA(1988) Aging-related skin changes: development and clinical meaning. *Geriatrics* **43**(4): 49–64

5

The measurement of interface pressure and its role in soft tissue breakdown

Iain Swain and Dan Bader

This chapter describes the effect of applied pressure on soft tissue and its possible role in the development of pressure ulcers. It concentrates on the quantification of the applied pressure at the patient–support interface and the limitations and variability of current techniques, measurement systems and data presentation. It then describes the effects of interface pressures at the tissue and cellular level, and attempts that have been made to describe and model the tissue mechanics. Finally, it sets a challenge to medical engineers to improve the present measurement systems and tissue models, thus increasing understanding, both clinically and at the cellular level, so that the incidence of pressure ulcers can be reduced.

There are a number of factors which can predispose an individual to a high risk of developing pressure ulcers. These can be divided into external factors including pressure, shear, time, temperature, humidity and their interactions, and internal factors which determine the level of loading tolerated by tissues before damage occurs (Guttmann, 1976). Some conditions affect the external factors by causing a loss of muscle bulk and tone, as in flaccid paraplegia, or by the weight loss associated with the latter stages of cancer. Others affect the external factors by increasing the time that pressure is applied without relief, such as in tetraplegia or in the later stages of multiple sclerosis where the patient is unable to move unaided. The internal factors can be affected by the underlying disease, such as diabetes or certain neurological conditions in which the tissues are more liable to be damaged by a given level of pressure.

There are only two ways associated with pressure in which a support surface can operate in order to reduce the probability of developing a pressure ulcer. First, there are static systems which seek to minimise the interface pressure by increasing the contact area, and second dynamic systems which produce an alternating action which subjects the tissues to periods of high pressure followed by periods of low pressure during which it is anticipated that the pressure is sufficiently low to enable blood flow to return.

The development of accurate pressure measuring systems is important in assessing such support systems. However, their exclusive use in determining risk of breakdown is critically dependent on a reliable indicator of safe pressure or band of pressures in association with time (Reswick and Rogers, 1976), which would be appropriate for all patients at risk. This remains a 'holy grail' for medical engineers involved in the prevention of pressure ulcers. Many attempts have been made to determine the minimal degree and duration of compression that will consistently produce tissue damage (Husain, 1953; Kosiak, 1961; Meijer *et al*, 1994). Typically, such values are extrapolated from *in-vivo* studies of human subjects or animal models in which soft tissues are compressed between external indenters and bony prominences within the body. Tissue damage is generally assessed from excised tissues or biopsies. These *in-vivo* studies lead to the description of qualitative risk curves which vary considerably because of differences in test specimens and experimental conditions, which are extremely difficult to control. What is undeniable, however, is that high pressures are sustainable for short time periods only, and, if maintained, they will lead to tissue breakdown.

Measurement of interface pressure

Pressure measurement systems can be used in two separate environments. First in a clinical setting, typically associated with a seating clinic, in which interface pressure is used as an adjunct to risk assessment as well as providing an aid to clinical prescription. It can also be used to give biofeedback to the patient to provide evidence of postural factors associated with pelvic obliquity, tilt and rotation and the efficacy of pressure relief regimens. Alternatively, it can be used in the laboratory to evaluate the relative performance of different pressure reduction systems under controlled conditions. Irrespective of how pressure-measuring systems are used, regular calibration must be undertaken.

Measurement of interface pressure is subject to great variability. There are differences between anatomical sites, between individuals and even when the sensor is kept on a single anatomical site on a given individual, there are differences caused by small changes in posture. There are also differences caused by clothing, the type of measurement system used and the interpretation of the data, ie. is the maximum or average pressure quoted or is some form of pressure index calculated? In order to compare products designed to reduce the incidence of pressure ulcers two alternative approaches have been adopted. First, indenters have been designed to replicate the loading patterns at the patient–support interface. Initially these were simple domed indenters (Bain, 1998) but, more recently, these have evolved into anthropomorphic mannequins with an internal skeleton covered by simulated soft tissues (Barnett and Shelton, 1997; Bain *et al*, 1999). Alternatively, meaningful data can be obtained from measurements on human subjects; but only if the experimental procedure is standardised, minimising the inherent variability. Each of these sources of variability will now be discussed in detail.

Variability resulting from measurement system

Any system designed to measure interface pressure will inherently have an effect on the very parameter that it is attempting to measure. There are a number of different systems that have been developed over the years ranging from single sensors, such as the original 28mm Scimedics system (Talley Medical, Romsey, Hampshire, UK) which needed to be manually inflated to record pressures, to systems like the 2000 element array (Tekscan Inc, Boston, MA, USA) which are capable of capturing data in real time and producing an image on a computer screen. Various researchers have advocated different systems, although to date there is no 'gold standard'.

Two main factors must be considered when measuring interface pressure:

1. The sensor must be correctly located under the relevant bony prominence.
2. The presence of the sensor must not introduce errors which would mask any difference between the support systems being evaluated.

As will be described, interface pressure has been shown to be significantly affected both by the positioning of the subject and by any object between the subject's skin and the support surface, particularly if that object is inflexible and cannot adapt to the shape of the patient–surface interface. In practice, these two factors are largely mutually exclusive as the large array systems have the advantage of many sensors, so that the point of maximum pressure can be determined easily, but have the disadvantage that if they are inflexible they will affect the surface, especially if the surface deforms in more than one dimension, as in the case of a low air loss or fluidised bead bed. If individual sensors are used then errors will be reduced if they are smaller than the area of interest, however, they will need to be accurately positioned to record the pressure exerted on the area of interest. If the sensor is larger than the area of interest it will act as an additional support, particularly if the sensor is inflated, and will therefore significantly change the patient–surface interface. Even if the sensor is of the correct size and type and is accurately placed, any readings taken are only a 'snap shot' of that particular situation and will vary with time and any change in posture of the patient.

There have been few reported comparisons of different pressure-measuring systems. Allen *et al* (1993; Allen and Ryan, 1993) looked at the repeatability and accuracy of the Talley SA500 Pressure Evaluator with both the 28mm and 100mm sensor pads (Talley Medical, Romsey, Hants, UK). This is an electropneumatic device in which the pressure needed to inflate an air sac is increased until two contacts on the internal faces of the air sac are broken. This pressure is then recorded as the interface pressure. They also evaluated the DIPE (Next Generation Co Inc, CA, USA) and found the Talley 28mm sensor was the most accurate. Ferguson-Pell and Cardill compared three systems, the Force Sensing Array (FSA) 225 sensors (Vista Medical Ltd, Winnipeg, Canada), the Tekscan 2064 sensors and the Talley Pressure Monitor (TPM) 96 sensors (Talley Medical, Romsey, Hampshire, UK). The TPM differs from the other two as it consists of small arrays of sensors as well as individual sensors which can be directly located on the skin surface. By contrast, the FSA and Tekscan are large arrays, typically 500mm x 500mm, which cover the whole area of interest. The authors found that the TPM was the most accurate, stable and reproducible of the systems tested but was limited in its ease of use, speed and data presentation (Ferguson-Pell and Cardi, 1993). The FSA was well rated in clinical applications but demonstrated pronounced hysteresis (±19%) and creep (4%). The Tekscan system also showed substantial hysteresis (±20%) and creep (19%) but was preferred by clinicians for its real time display capabilities, resolution and display options.

Gyi *et al* (1998) undertook a detailed critique of the TPM, a more recent derivative of the Oxford Pressure Monitor (Bader and Hawken, 1986), which examines the pressure–flow characteristics of the air needed to inflate a small air sac. This has been shown to give good correlation with the Talley SA 500 (Norman *et al*, 1995). These authors identified a major disadvantage of this system in that it did not give readings in real time as it samples one sensor element approximately every second and therefore each sensor is sampled only every 90 seconds if all 96 sensors are connected. Other findings were that the system was improved if the sensor elements were more tightly packed and that errors could occur if the sensors were placed on a curved surface, although the errors were small if the radius of curvature was less than 20mm. In addition, if only 75% of the sensor face was covered then the reading obtained was 82% of the correct value. The authors are unaware of any other evaluations of this type and it is clear that similar studies are required to quantify errors associated with the measurement of interface pressure.

Methods of displaying and analysing the data

Whatever measurement system is used, the data must be collected and presented in an appropriate form. If used in the clinical environment the data have to be interpreted easily both by clinicians and patients, whereas in research the raw data are necessary for statistical analysis. The simplest presentation involves quoting an instantaneous value of interface pressure but this could prove unreliable if the measurement procedure was not sufficiently rigorous or the value was not representative of the measurement over time. Thus, such a value could prove harmful if given too much clinical significance. It could be argued that the way the data is presented should be related to the support system being evaluated. Therefore data presentation would vary depending whether measurements are made on a static system, a dynamic or alternating system or whether the support surfaces demonstrate any inherent hysteresis or creep, as in the case of viscoelastic foams.

If the information is required for clinical use or patient education, then the graphical representation of the interface pressures might be more important than the absolute accuracy. The display of data needs to be in real time and easy to interpret so that both patients and non-technical clinical staff can observe the effects of movement, changing support surfaces, etc. To do this in the clinical environment necessitates that the system is easy to use and that an overall picture of the patient–surface interface can be displayed at a glance, thus avoiding the need for the accurate placement of sensors. This application would be ideally served by using multisensor arrays, such as the Tekscan or FSA.

For comparison between two or more commercial products much greater care is needed to ensure that the measurement system and the way the results are presented do not distort any differences between the products. The simplest case is that of comparing two static systems. First, the experimental procedure has to be designed and standardised to minimise errors by controlling position and by taking multiple readings to ensure that the sensors are directly positioned under the points of interest (Swain *et al*, 1993; Swain *et al*, 1994; Swain *et al*, 1995; Swain and Peters, 1997; Hobson, 1992; Peters and Swain, 1998; Bar, 1988). In addition, falsely high readings caused by factors such as creases in the sensors must be avoided. Once the data have been collected the majority of researchers have used the maximum interface pressure under the area of interest as the parameter to be compared in any statistical analysis (Meijer *et al*, 1994; Bain, 1998; Swain *et al*, 1993; Swain *et al*, 1994; Swain *et al*, 1995; Swain and Peters, 1997; Hobson, 1992; Swain *et al*, 1992; Rondolf-Klym and Langamo, 1993; Brienza and Karg, 1998; Kernozek and Lewin, 1998; Brienza *et al*, 1996) although others have calculated an average pressure over a selected area (Kernozek *et al*, 1996). It is noticeable that those authors who have used an average pressure find less difference between rival products. Nevertheless, even when maximum values are used, few trials report differences between product performance which are statistically significant at the 5% level.

Two studies have chosen to define other parameters calculated from the data generated by multisensor arrays in an attempt to give an overall impression of the relative performance of different support surfaces. Patel *et al* (1993) calculated a pressure index which was based on threshold levels, whereas Shelton *et al* (1998) calculated a pressure index based on statistical analysis.

The possibility of presenting the data in different forms is far greater when dynamic systems such as alternating pressure mattresses are being considered, as by their very nature they will exert periods of high pressure followed by periods of low pressure. The most commonly quoted parameters are maximum, minimum and average pressures but these provide little indication as to the length of time that the pressure is at a lower value. This has led a number of researchers (Bar, 1988; Rithalia and Gonsalkorale, 1998) reporting the amount of time the interface pressure is above or below a certain threshold, most conveniently displayed in histogram form. Although there is still considerable debate over what constitutes a safe interface pressure, there is to date no consensus.

Given that a suitable method can be found to analyse and present the data, all the above have only considered a subject in a defined posture, which is not representative of real life. In particular, an individual in a wheelchair is constantly changing their position both in the short term as they propel and in the longer term because of their activities of daily living. Of the few studies to have considered this, Bar (1988) produced a pressure–time histogram over a prolonged sitting period and both Dabnichki and Taktak (1998) and Kernozek and Lewin (1998) considered the variation of interface pressure during the wheelchair push cycle. The former study indicated that the interface pressures were speed dependant and could be increased by as much as 125% when compared to the situation at rest (Dabnichki and Taktak, 1998).

Inter-subject variability

As pressure is force per unit area it is obvious that the shape of a subject will have an effect on the interface pressure. The shape of the subject will depend on the skeleton, the quantity, tone and shape of the musculature and the amount of subcutaneous fat. However, from *Figure 5.1* it can be seen that there is no trend evident between a subject's weight and the interface pressure. This finding has also been confirmed in other trials (Allen *et al*, 1993). In addition, no trend has been shown between the interface pressure and the subject's build which can be characterised by the body mass index (BMI = weight/height^2), as illustrated in *Figure 5.2*. The effect that an individual's anatomy has on interface pressure is therefore much more subtle and even individuals with very similar body types can exhibit quite different interface pressures. This can be demonstrated well from the baseline data on the standard King's Fund mattress obtained by one of the authors in both Department of Health funded and commercial trials (Norman *et al*, 1995; Swain *et al*, 1993; Swain *et al*, 1994; Swain *et al*, 1995; Swain and Peters, 1997). A minimum of twenty readings made on different days have been used to calculate these means and standard deviations.

For example, subject A who is 1.57m tall with a BMI of 23.6 has a mean interface pressure under the sacrum when semi-recumbent in bed of 61.9±9.2mmHg (8.3±1.2kPa), whereas subject B (height 1.57m, BMI 23.1) has an interface pressure of 86.4±12.2mmHg (11.5±1.6kPa). This effect is even more marked when the heels are considered as there is great variation between individuals' anatomy and again, on the standard King's Fund mattress, variations from a mean of 107±22.6mmHg (14.3±3.1kPa) to a mean of 231±46.6mmHg (30.8±6.2kPa) have been seen. Clearly some individuals have smaller, more bony heels than others and as the contact area of a heel on a relatively non-conforming surface is so small, any slight difference in contact area will have a major effect on the interface pressure. Errors in measurement will also increase as the placement of the sensor is far more critical if the contact area is small.

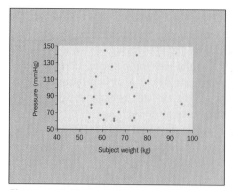

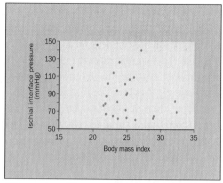

Figure 5.1: The variability of interface pressure with the weight of the subject. From Swain and Peters, 1997

Figure 5.2: The variability of interface pressure with body mass index of the subject. From Swain and Peters, 1997

Therefore the range of interface pressures on various anatomical sites vary widely with the subjects' underlying anatomy and, in the authors' experience, it is not possible to predict the interface pressures from the person's body type.

Interface pressures were measured on the King's Fund mattress at the most common locations for pressure ulcers by one of the authors (*Table 5.1*). These readings were made using elderly ambulant volunteers and were obtained from readings made during the production of the Department of Health evaluation reports PS1, PS2, PS3, PS4, PS5 and MDA/97/2015,16,17,18,20,32 and from fifteen years' consultancy work for a great number of companies.

Table 5.1: Interface pressures at common pressure locations	
Sacrum when semi-recumbent, backrest at 45°	62–107 mmHg (8.3–14.3 kPa)
Trochanter, side lying, hips and knees at 60°	61–156 mmHg (8.1–20.8 kPa)
Heels	107–213 mmHg (14.3–28.4 kPa)
Ischials when sitting on a 3-inch standard cushion	60–146 mmHg (8.0–19.5 kPa)

Variability resulting from anatomical location and patient position

The human body is not a homogenous structure and the interface pressure will vary depending on the shape of the underlying bony structure at the point of interest, the amount of subcutaneous tissue covering that bone and the weight being supported. High pressure points will either be areas such as the heels when lying supine, where there is a small contact area, or the buttocks when sitting, where there is a large load combined with underlying bony prominences, the ischial tuberosities. If this contact area is further reduced by extensive loss of subcutaneous tissue, then the pressures will increase. When lying supine, a person with normal pathology will have much lower interface pressures under the buttocks because the load is distributed over a larger area and as the pelvis is rotated, compared to sitting, there are no obvious bony prominences in contact with the support surface. In this position more pressure will be exerted on the sacrum, particularly if the person is semi-recumbent. The person's posture will have a marked effect on the areas subjected to the highest pressures. For example, a person sitting in a slumped position in a chair will often have the highest pressures recorded under the sacrum rather than under the ischial tuberosities.

When comparing different products, it is essential to ensure repeatable positioning of the subjects, as failure to do so can lead to errors which are greater than the underlying differences between the products. This is best demonstrated by the results obtained during the Department of Health trial on wheelchair cushions (Swain and Peters, 1997; Peters and Swain, 1997). In this trial, it was found that adjusting the footrest height made more difference to the interface pressure, as indicated in *Figure 5.3*, than changing from the best cushions tested to the worst. By changing the footrest height in twelve subjects the mean interface pressure increased twofold from 65mmHg to 130mmHg (8.7–17.3kPa), whereas changing the type of cushion from the best to the worst saw an increase in interface pressure from 71 to 128mmHg (9.5–17.1kPa).

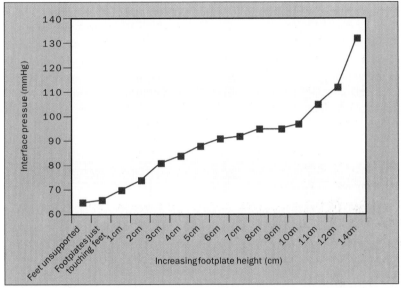

Figure 5.3: The variability of interface pressure with footplate height for the seated subject. From Swain and Peters, 1997

This variability is also reported by other researchers. Koo *et al* (1996) found that interface pressure in seated patients could increase from 88 to 146mmHg (11.7–19.5kPa) on a Roho cushion and from 106 to 221mmHg (14.1–29.5kPa) on a polyurethane foam cushion, as the patient varied his/her position in the chair from leaning forward to leaning to the right. This indicates that the more conforming the cushion, the less effect posture has on interface pressure. Hobson (1992) also found that posture and body orientation had a profound effect on body–seat interface variables and that posture is a factor which deserves increased research and clinical attention.

Variability caused by underlying pathology

Expediency often requires that interface pressure readings are undertaken on healthy, young adult volunteers, often students, despite the fact that the vast majority of people at risk of pressure ulcers are elderly or those with chronic diseases, illness or disabilities. In those at risk there will not only be a change in shape at the patient–support interface as a result of loss in muscle tone, but the skin will often have inferior mechanical properties and the body may be less able to adapt to the effects of pressure as a result of the underlying pathology. This is particularly the case if the underlying disease affects the normal circulatory control system, such as in multiple sclerosis and spinal bifida.

Of the few studies to compare the interface pressure of different groups, Brienza and Karg (1998) showed that the type of cushion had a greater effect on subjects with spinal cord injury than it did with the elderly, but suggested that more research was still needed. Hobson (1992) also noted that people with spinal cord injuries exhibited interface pressures between 6% and 46% higher than a control group of normal subjects.

One of the most unexpected findings to emerge from the Department of Health report PS432 was that, irrespective of the type of cushion, the interface pressures measured on the four different groups of subjects (elderly, cardiovascular accident, spastic paraplegics and flaccid paraplegics) were always ranked in the same order, with the elderly volunteers exhibiting the lowest pressures and the flaccid paraplegics the highest, as shown in *Figure 5.4*. It can also be seen that for the elderly subjects the choice of cushion made comparatively little difference. By contrast, in the flaccid paraplegic group there was much greater variation and therefore the choice of the cushion made far more difference to the interface pressure.

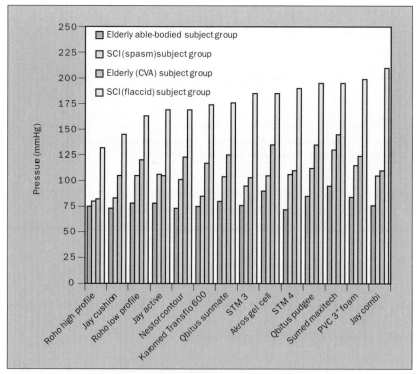

Figure 5.4: The variability of interface pressure on a range of cushions with four subject groups. From Swain and Peters, 1997
VCA = cardiovascular accident; SCI = spinal cord injury

Variability resulting from other factors such as clothing

A static support surface is required to conform to the shape of the body so that the load can be distributed over a larger area, hence reducing the interface pressure. In a dynamic support surface, such as an alternating pressure mattress, it is essential that nothing affects the alternating action so that when a given cell is deflated, the interface pressure is sufficiently low to enable blood flow to return to normal levels before the next period of high pressure when the cell is reinflated. In both types of systems the properties of any covering materials between the foam, air or gel of the cushion and the subject's skin will affect the interface pressure. If the covering material is too tight and inflexible then it will tend to hammock across the support surface, preventing deformation of the underlying core in static systems and negating the alternating action in dynamic systems. This was demonstrated in PS115 when it was found that by changing the cover on a standard King's Fund foam mattress, the pressure could be decreased by an average of 13% if a one-way stretch cover was used, or increased by 48% if a heavier, non-stretch material was fitted.

For this reason the majority of support surfaces in current use have a two-way stretch cover to prevent hammocking. The majority also have a vapour-permeable cover which is claimed to reduce the amount of perspiration. The effect of the covering material is also important when advising the wheelchair or chairbound patient on the choice of clothing. Stretchy sports clothing will be far better for the patient than heavy materials like denim, which are non-conforming and usually have thick seams and rivets in support areas.

The effects of applied pressure

Despite the problems described above, interface pressures at the tissue surface can be measured. However, their relationship with the interstitial stresses (and strains) within the tissues has rarely been explored. This is, in part, because of the requirement for an invasive measurement. Of the few studies, Sangeorzan *et al* (1989) noted that the two values were not equivalent and were highly dependent on the nature of the intervening soft tissues. Thus, the thickness, tone and mechanical integrity of subcutaneous tissues and the proximity of bony prominences will influence this relationship.

An investigation of subjects during surgical procedures examined the response of tissues adjacent to the lateral aspect of the proximal thigh. Results indicated that skin interface pressures were dissipated within the depth of the tissues, resulting in reduced internal stresses (Bader and White, 1998). Indeed, linear models of the data suggested interstitial stresses ranging between 29% and 40% of the applied interface pressures, as illustrated in *Figure 5.5*. This highlights the protective nature of tissues to attenuate the effects of sustained pressure. It is interesting to note that, in many cases, the interstitial pressures exceeded 32mmHg (5.3kPa), a value often used in clinical practice. This value was based on the measured pressure in the skin capillaries within the nail folds (Landis, 1930) and thus represents a measure of localised interstitial pressure not relevant to areas at risk of pressure-induced damage. Its use is totally inappropriate as a threshold value for interface pressures at load-bearing sites.

A knowledge of the nature of the stresses occurring at the interface is essential in the assessment of the potential damage to soft tissues. It is well known that body tissues can support high levels of hydrostatic pressure, with equal components in all directions, with no resulting tissue distortion. This may be illustrated in the case of deep sea divers, who are regularly exposed to hydrostatic pressures in excess of 750mmHg (100kPa) for prolonged periods with no deleterious effects to the soft tissues. However, if the pressures are non-uniform then localised tissue damage can result. This is the case in many of the situations in which the body interfaces externally with load-carrying devices, such as the provision of support surfaces for wheelchair and chair-bound individuals and at the stump–socket interface of lower limb prostheses.

Pressure changes in the environment may transmit their effects to living cells in a number of ways. For example, it has been well established that relatively high pressures applied hydrostatically are necessary in order to produce significant changes in physiological functions (Cattel, 1936). For example, hydrostatic pressures in excess of 5×10^5 mmHg (70MPa) are required to produce irreversible changes in most forms of protoplasm. However, when the pressure is applied locally there is an initial displacement of the fluid portion of the cell, followed by an irreversible disorganisation of the more rigid structures. These effects are more pronounced at the periphery of the compression area where the pressure gradient, and therefore distribution, is at a maximum. For example, a pressure of only 200mmHg (26.7kPa) applied directly for a few minutes was found to be sufficient to inhibit nerve conduction (Cattel, 1936).

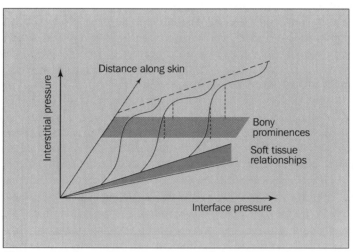

Figure 5.5: Schematic representation of the relationship between interface pressure and interstitial pressure at different tissue locations. From Sangeorzan *et al*, 1989; Bader and White, 1998

Events at the tissue level

The mechanical environment may be sufficient to impair the integrity of the local blood supply and lymphatic circulation. Impairment of the former will limit the availability of oxygen to the localised tissues, while lymphatic impairment results in an accumulation of toxic intracellular materials in the tissues (Bader, 1990). If the interface conditions are prolonged, cell necrosis will follow, leading to possible tissue breakdown and the development of pressure ulcers.

If the pressure is relieved periodically, higher pressures can be tolerated for longer periods. This forms the basis of pressure relief regimens, which involve regular turning, lift-off from the support surface and use of alternating pressure support systems. The nature of the tissue recovery is determined by the resilience of the specific tissues and the tissue structures, including the blood and lymph vessels. The soft tissues exhibit viscoelastic behaviour and thus the nature of the recovery will depend upon the rate and time of loading as well as its magnitude. Short-term loading generally produces elastic deformation with minimal creep and rapid elastic recovery, whereas long-term loading results in marked creep and requires significant time for complete tissue recovery (Bader, 1990). Indeed, it has been well established that tissue damage is often apparent following prolonged loading even at relatively low level pressure intensities (Reswick and Rogers, 1976). Any significant period of loading will result in vascular occlusion. On load removal, there will be a period of increased blood flow through the tissues which had been ischaemic. This phenomenon, termed reactive hyperaemia, is a consequence of a local regulatory mechanism whereby the arterioles are dilated and the resistance to blood flow is reduced. This mechanism may be impaired in chronic disease states. It has been suggested that this reperfusion of blood and transport of nutrients can result in a cascade of harmful effects, including the over-production and release of oxygen-derived free radicals (Pretto, 1991; Peirce *et al*, 2000). This establishes the so-called ischaemic/reperfusion injury, which have been implicated in the damage of many tissues and organs.

Individual differences in the load-bearing capacity of soft tissue composite largely influence the onset of pressure ulcers, because of predisposing factors such as age or physical wellbeing. Although individual effects can be examined, it is difficult to assess their combined influence on pressure ulcer development. Additionally, the relative susceptibility of individual tissue layers to pressure-induced damage is variable. Indeed, some studies have shown that muscle tissue is highly susceptible to localised compression, eventually leading to tissue degeneration in the form of a deep pressure ulcer which progresses towards the skin surface (Daniel *et al*, 1982; Nola and Vistnes, 1980).

Events at the cellular level

Tissue degeneration starts at the cellular level and is characterised by nuclear pyknosis and an early disintegration of the contractile proteins in the cells, followed by inflammatory reactions and tissue necrosis (Kosiak, 1961; Nola and Vistnes, 1980; Caplan *et al*, 1988). Although it is clear that both the magnitude and duration of compression affect cellular breakdown, the underlying mechanisms whereby tissue compression results in cell damage are poorly understood. Theories on impaired perfusion and transport of nutrients and metabolic waste products across the cell membrane can only partly explain the onset of tissue damage and have, to date, not been fully verified (Daniel *et al*, 1982; Dodd and Gross, 1991; Krouskop, 1983; Vohra and McCollum, 1994).

It has been hypothesised that sustained deformation of the muscle cells in the tissue plays an additional role in this process. Cell deformation triggers a variety of effects which may be involved in early cell damage, such as local membrane stresses which may lead to buckling and bursting of the membrane, volume changes, and modifications of cytoskeletal organisation affecting its integrity (Petersen *et al*, 1982).

In addition, changes in the mechanical and chemical environment of the cell may induce further damage. A contribution of cell deformation to mechanotransduction, ie. the process by which muscle cells detect and respond to their mechanical environment, which influences cell damage and adaptation, might be expected in the presence of compressive strains.

An *in-vitro* system involving cultured muscle cells has been developed, consisting of cultured muscle cells embedded in agarose gel. This system enables improved control of experimental conditions and offers the potential for reproducible, well-characterised specimens (Bouten *et al*, 2001). This system has demonstrated that a longer compression period will lead to an increased proportion of muscle cells being damaged (Bouten *et al*, 1999). Initial results, as illustrated in *Figure 6.6*, confirm that both the level of applied compression and its duration are key factors in determining cell viability in the model system. This finding is analogous to the earlier observations with human subjects by Reswick and Rogers (1976) and suggests that: 'prolonged compression of cells leading to loss of viability can represent a key element in the development of pressure sores'.

Tissue mechanics and modelling

The compression characteristics of the soft tissues influence their susceptibility to the breakdown process. Areas at particular risk include the sacrum and the ischium which have minimal soft tissue compliance over bony prominences. Under external loading high interstitial stresses and strains will be developed within these areas. These conditions may occlude the blood and lymphatic vessels, although local vessel architecture may ultimately determine site susceptibility. The overall properties of the skin and soft tissue as a composite in compression have received relatively little attention. Bader and Bowker (1983) used a counterbalanced beam to load the skin and soft tissue composite. They determined the estimated values of compressive stiffness derived from tissue recovery, which were on average 25% higher than those derived from tissue indentation tests. This was evident for subjects of different ages and from differing tissue sites. In a more recent study, an indentation method was used to examine the effects of muscular activities on the mechanical properties of stump soft tissues on amputees (Mak *et al*, 1994).

An alternative approach to measure stiffness is to examine the change in shape of loaded soft tissues compared to their unloaded shape using ultrasound (Kadaba *et al*, 1986; Ophir *et al*, 1999). In particular, the recent development of elastography, associated with the ultrasonic imaging of tissues, may provide a reliable means of estimating materials' properties under compressive loading in both the research and clinical setting (Ophir *et al*, 1999). Magnetic resonance imaging techniques have also been used to visualise soft tissues; from these images, measurements of tissue deformation were recorded at various applied compressive loads (Reger *et al*, 1990). A clear distinction was demonstrated between the mechanical response of healthy tissues adjacent to the ischial tuberosities of a normal subject compared to the atrophied soft tissues of an age-matched paraplegic with flaccid paralysis. The latter tissues were observed to be more distorted under load, suggesting an increased risk of tissue trauma.

The increased propensity for paraplegics with flaccid paralysis to develop pressure ulcers was also recorded in an extensive clinical study (Noble, 1982). A mechanism was suggested by a study examining the viability of loaded tissues, as assessed by transcutaneous gas monitoring, on a population of spinal cord-injured patients (Bogie *et al*, 1995). Paraplegic subjects with reduced muscle tone and a progressive loss of muscle bulk throughout the rehabilitation phase, in particular, demonstrated a compromised viability during periods of sitting. The atrophic changes will reduce the amount of soft tissue surrounding the arterial capillary bed and thus increase the effect of the applied pressure. In contrast, the physical characteristics of the soft tissue in the spinal cord injured subject with spastic paralysis are considered to be similar to a normal subject. Tissue viability under applied loads at the seating interface was generally observed to be improved in subjects with a degree of muscle tone below the level of the lesion. Thus, muscle bulk and blood flow are greater in subjects with upper motor neuron lesions compared to those with lower motor neuron lesions. The presence of spasm means that muscle bulk and blood flow are partially maintained despite the absence of useful functional movement.

Current status

Although it is known that applied pressure is a major causative factor in pressure aetiology, the exact mechanism and even the level of pressure required is unknown. In addition, its associated effects with parameters such as tangential forces and interface temperatures have still to be examined. This has not been helped by the lack of both understanding and scientific rigour in the measurement and reporting of interface pressure in the literature, which has lead to a polarisation of views. On the one hand, there is a degree of scepticism associated with the usefulness of measuring interface pressures and, on the other hand, an over-reliance on its use to prescribe support surfaces.

An alternative approach would be to analyse the transmission of forces across the patient interface. These forces and resulting stress and strain distributions are complex in nature. This is reflected in the relatively few attempts at producing mathematical (Dabnichki and Taktak, 1998; Bouten *et al*, 1999; Murphy and Bennett, 1971; Chow and Odell, 1978; Todd and Thacker, 1994) and empirical (Candadai and Reddy, 1992) solutions to the problem. A description of the mathematical approach is beyond the scope of this chapter, but it is worth noting that the more recent models incorporating non-linear and hyperelastic behaviour are more realistic than the more traditional approaches, which have assumed that the soft tissues exhibit linearly elastic and isotropic properties.

The measurement and understanding of the effects of interface pressure, both clinically and at the cellular level, provides a challenge to medical engineers. Meeting this challenge will require ingenuity combined with meticulous experimental technique to capitalise on the improvements in sensor technology, which for the first time have enabled measurements to be made over long periods of time and hence allowed a more complete understanding of pressure ulcer aetiology. This, in turn, will provide meaningful information that can be presented in a format that may enable clinicians to reduce the incidence of ulcers.

Key points

⌘ This chapter reviews the often complex and confusing subject of interface pressure measurement. Understanding the forces applied to the skin and soft tissue lies at the heart of our understanding of pressure ulceration.

⌘ Understanding interface pressure and how it can be modified by both subject and environmental factors will help enhance our awareness of the mechanical forces on the body, its tissues and constitutent cells.

⌘ Over several years understanding interface pressure has become confused by the conflicting marketing claims made to support pressure redistributing projects. This review reclaims the science behind and appropriate interpretation of interface pressure data.

References

Allen V, Ryan DW, Murray A (1993) Repeatability of subject/bed interface pressure measurements. *J Biomed Engineering* **15**: 329–32

Allen V, Ryan DW, Lomax N, Murray A (1993) Accuracy of interface pressure measurement systems. *J Biomed Engineering* **15**: 344–8

Bader DL, Hawken MB (1986) Pressure distribution under the ischium of the normal subject. *J Biomed Engineering* **8**: 353–7

Bader DL, Bowker P (1983) Mechanical characteristics of skin and underlying tissues *in vivo*. *Biomaterials* **4**: 305–8

Bader DL (1990) The recovery characteristics of soft tissues following repeated loading. *J Rehabil Res Dev* **27**(2): 141–50

Bader DL, White SH (1998) The viability of soft tissues in elderly subjects undergoing hip surgery. *Age Ageing* **27**: 217–21

Bain DS (1998) Testing the effectiveness of patient support systems: the importance of indenter geometry. *J Tissue Viability* **8**(1): 15–17

Bain DS, Scales JT, Nicholson GP (1999) A new method of assessing the mechanical properties of patient support systems (PSS) using a phantom. A preliminary report. *Medical Engineering and Physics* **21**(5): 293–301

Bar CA (1988) The response of tissue to applied pressure. PhD thesis. University of Wales, Cardiff

Barnett RI, Shelton FE (1997) Measurement of support surface efficiency. *Adv Wound Care* **10**(7): 21–29

Bogie KM, Nuseibeh I, Bader DL (1995) Early progressive changes in tissue viability in the seated spinal cord injured subject. *Paraplegia* **33**: 141–7

Bouten CVC, Boboom EMH, Oomens CWJ (1999) The aetiology of pressure sores: A tissue and cell mechanics approach. In: van der Woulde LHV, ed. *Biomedical Aspects of Manual Wheelchair Propulsion*. IOS Press, Amsterdam: 52–62

Bouten CVC, Knight MM, Lee DA, Bader DL (2001) Compressive deformation and damage of muscle cell subpopulations in a model system. *Ann Biomechanical Engineering* **29**: 153–63

Brienza DM, Karg PE, Brubaker CE (1996) Seat cushion design for elderly wheelchair users based on minimisation of soft tissue deformation using stiffness and pressure measurements. *IEEE Transactions in Biomedical Engineering* **4**(4): 320–7

Brienza DM, Karg PE (1998) Seat cushion optimisation: a comparison of interface pressure and tissue stiffness characteristics for spinal cord injured and elderly patients. *Arch Phys Med Rehabil* **79**: 388–94

Candadai RS, Reddy NP (1992) Stress distribution in a physical buttock model: effect of simulated bone geometry. *J Biomech* **25**: 1403–11

Caplan A, Carlson B, Faulkner J, Fischman D, Garrett W (1988) Skeletal muscle. In: Woo SL-Y, Buckwalter JA, ed. Injury and repair of the musculoskeletal soft tissues. *Am Academy of Orthopaedic Surgeons*: 213–91

Cattel M (1936) The physiological effects of pressure. *Biol Rev* **11**: 441–74

Chow WW, Odell EI (1978) Deformations and stresses in soft body tissues of a sitting person. *J Biomech Eng* **100**: 79–87

Dabnichki P, Taktak D (1998) Pressure variation under the ischial tuberosity during a push cycle. *Med Eng Phys* **20**: 242–56

Daniel RK, Priest DL, Wheatley DC (1982) Etiologic factors in pressure sores: an experimental model. *Arch Phys Med Rehabil* **62**: 492–8

Dodd KT, Gross DR (1991) Three-dimensional tissue deformation in subcutaneous tissues overlying bony prominences may help to explain external load transfer to the interstitium. *J Biomechanics* **24**: 11–19

Ferguson-Pell M, Cardi MD (1993) Prototype development and comparative evaluation of wheelchair pressure mapping systems. *Assistive Technology* **5**(2): 78–91

Guttmann L (1976) The prevention and treatment of pressure sores. In: Kenedi RM, Cowden JM, Scales JT, eds. *Bedsore Biomechanics*. Macmillan, London: 153–9

Gyi DE, Porter JM, Robertson NKB (1998) Seat pressure measurement technologies: considerations for their evaluation. *Applied Ergonomics* **27**: 85–91

Hobson DA (1992) Comparative effects of posture on pressure and shear at the body seat interface. *J Rehabil Res Dev* **29**: 21–31

Husain T (1953) An experimental study of some pressure effects on tissues, with reference to the bed sore problem. *J Pathology Bacteriology* : 347–58

Kadaba MP, Ferguson-Pell MW, Palmieri V, Cochran GVB (1986) Ultrasound mapping of the buttock-cushion interface contour. *Arch Phys Med Rehabil* **23**: 33–9

Kernozek TW, Breyen P, Piccanatto B (1996) Influence of hip and ankle position on the seat pressure distribution disabled elderly. *Physical Therapy* **76**(5): S22

Kernozek TW, Lewin JE (1998) Seat interface pressure of individuals with paraplegia: influence of dynamic wheelchair locomotion compared with static seated measurements. *Arch Phys Med Rehabil* **79**: 313–16

Koo TKK, Mak AFT, Lee YL (1996) Posture effects on seating interface biomechanics; comparison between two seating cushions. *Arch Phys Med Rehabil* **77**: 40–7

Kosiak M (1961) Etiology of decubitus ulcers. *Arch Physical Medicine and Rehabilitation* **42**: 19–29

Krouskop TA (1983) A synthesis of the factors that contribute to pressure sore formation. *Med Hypotheses* **11**: 255–67

Landis EM (1930) Micro-injection studies of capillary blood pressure in human skin. *Heart* **15**: 209–28

Mak AFT, Liu GHW, Lee SY (1994) Biomechanical assessment of below-knee residual limb tissue. *J Rehabil Res Dev* **31**(3):188–98

Meijer JH, Germs PH, Schneider H, Ribbe MW (1994) Susceptibility to decubitus ulcer formation. *Arch Phys Med Rehabil* **75**: 318–23

Murphy EF, Bennett L (1971) Transferring load to flesh, Parts 1 and 2. *Bull Prosthetic Res* **10-16**: 38–63

Noble (1982) Pressure sores and spinal injuries. In: Noble P, ed. *Prevention of Pressure Sores in Persons with Spinal Cord Injury*. World Rehabilitation Fund Inc, New York: 43–55

Nola GT, Vistnes LM (1980) Differential response of skin and muscle in the experimental production of pressure sores. *Plast Reconstr Surg* **66**: 728–33

Norman D, Dunford C, Swain ID (1995) Assessment of support surfaces – Mistral Mattress and Bodipillo Overlay. *J Tissue Viability* **5**(4): 115–17

Ophir J, Alam SK, Garra B, Kallel F, Konofagou E, Krouskop T, Varghese T (1999) Elastography: ultrasonic estimation and imaging of the elastic properties of tissues. *Proc Inst Mech Eng* **Part H 213**: 203–33

Patel UH, Jones JT, Babbs CF, Bourland JD, Graber G (1993) The evaluation of five specialist support surfaces by use of a pressure sensitive mat. *Decubitus* **6**(3): 28–37Reswick JB, Rogers JE (1976) Experience at Rancho Los Amigos Hospital with devices and techniques to prevent pressure sores. In: Kenedi RM, Cowden JM, Scales JT, eds. *Bedsore Biomechanics*. Macmillan, London: 301–10

Peirce SM, Skalak TC, Rodheheaver GT (2000) Ischaemic-reperfusion injury in chronic pressure ulcer formation: A skin model in the rat. *Wound Repair Regeneration* **8**: 68–76

Peters E, Swain ID (1997) *Evaluation of Wheelchair Cushions, Static and Dynamic. PS4*. Medical Devices Agency, Nowich, Department of Health

Peters E, Swain ID (1998) *Evaluation of pressure relieving ward chairs, PS5*. Medical Devices Agency, Norwich, Department of Health

Petersen NO, McConnaughey WB, Elson EL (1982) Dependence of locally measured cellular deformability on position on the cell, temperature, and cytochalasin B. *Proc Natl Acad Sci* **79**: 5327–31

Pretto EA (1991) Reperfusion injury of the liver. *Transplant Proc* **23**: 1912–14

Reger SI, McGovern TF, Chung KC (1990) Biomechanics of tissue distortion and stiffness by magnetic resonance imaging. In: Bader DL, ed. *Pressure Sores — clinical practice and scientific approach*. Macmillan, Basingstoke: 177–90

Rithalia SVS, Gonsalkorale M (1998) Assessment of alternating air mattresses using a time based interface pressure threshold technique. *J Rehabil Res* **35**(2): 225–30

Rondolf-Klym LM, Langamo D (1993) Relationship between body weight, body position, support surface and tissue interface pressure at the sacrum. *Decubitus* **6**(1): 22–30

Sangeorzan BJ, Harrington RM, Wyss CR, Czerniecki JM, Matsen FA (1989) Circulation and mechanical response of skin to loading. *J Orthop Res* **7**: 425–31

Shelton F, Barnett R, Meyer E (1998) Full-length interface pressure testing as a method for performance evaluation of clinical support surfaces. *Applied Ergonomics* **29**(6): 491–7

Swain ID, Nash RSW, Robertson JC (1992) Objective assessment of the Nimbus and Pegasus Airwave Mattresses. *J Tissue Viability* **2**(2): 43–5

Swain ID, Stacey PO, Dunford CE, Nichols R (1993) *Evaluation, PS1 Foam Mattresses*. Medical Devices Directorate, Norwich, Department of Health

Swain ID, Stacey PO, Dunford CE, Nichols R (1994) *Evaluation, PS2 Static Overlays*. Medical Devices Agency, Norwich, Department of Health

Swain ID, Stacey PO, Dunford CE, Nichols R (1995) *Evaluation, PS3 Alternating Pressure Overlays*. Medical Devices Agency, Norwich, Department of Health

Swain ID, Peters E (1997) *The effects of posture body mass index and wheelchair adjustment on interface pressures. Evaluation Report MDA/97/20.* Medical Devices Agency, Norwich, Department of Health

Todd BA, Thacker JG (1994) Three-dimensional computer model of the human buttocks, in vivo. *J Rehabil Res Dev* **31**(2): 111–19

Vohra RK, McCollum CN (1994) Pressure sores. *Br Med J* **309**: 853–7

Section III:
Prevention: what works and what doesn't

This section introduces appraisals of the effectiveness of pressure ulcer prevention interventions. Starting with the simplest intervention — manual repositioning of patients — the evidence is sifted and the multiple gaps in our current knowledge exposed. The chapter then turns to pressure redistributing support surfaces with an example of how laboratory evaluation can provide indirect pointers towards potential differences in their clinical effectiveness. However, the clinical outcome we are interested in (prevention of a pressure ulcer) may be influenced by many factors where formal randomised controlled trials often exclude these important factors in an attempt to recruit homogeneous patient populations. The third chapter in this section describes a large study that collected data upon what happened to patients in UK hospitals; with over 2500 subjects recruited the data offers potential for detailed exploration of the risk factors that truly make people vulnerable to pressure ulcer development. Finally, in this section a thoughtful chapter provides consideration as to whether we place too much importance upon support surfaces when tackling pressure ulcer prevention. This is a challenging debate — for almost twenty years pressure ulcer prevention in the United Kingdom has effectively equated with the identification of what should be the appropriate mattress for that patient (and maybe a seat cushion also!). What if this approach was a blind alley? Twenty years after the explosion of support surface dissemination in UK healthcare, there still is no evidence that the more sophisticated (and expensive) interventions such as alternating pressure mattresses are more effective than high-quality foam mattresses (NICE, 2003). This gap requires to be closed with either multiple studies confirming the value of sophisticated support surfaces or will we eventually abandon this route towards pressure ulcer prevention? It is important to reflect that a lack of evidence does not automatically mean a lack of effect but simply notes that rigorous studies have not yet been reported. If we are to offer effective prevention then major gaps in our understanding of the effect of common interventions could be seen as being unacceptable.

6

Manual repositioning: turning patients and reducing risk

Miles E Maylor

This chapter considers patient turning, the place of risk assessment and 'stepping down'. A warning note is sounded in that comfort does not necessarily equate with safety. Risk assessment scales have been linked with the selection of equipment, but it will be suggested that this is both misleading and unnecessarily complicated. What do staff do in the face of limited resources or when faced with the question of whether to keep someone on pressure-reducing equipment when it might no longer be necessary in order to prevent pressure ulceration? In other words, how can one rationally justify a strategy that appears to be protective but may be a waste of money or, worse, harmful to a process of rehabilitation? Some principles will be suggested as to how to approach difficult choices.

Turning and pressure reduction

There is a complex relationship between patient movement and the incidence of pressure ulcers (Maylor, 2001a). Regular repositioning of patients to redistribute pressure has been advocated by several sources (Norton, 1975; Agency for Health Care Policy and Research, 1994 [reviewed 2000]; Kanj *et al*, 1998; Rycroft-Malone, 2000). There is a consensus among UK 'experts' that individuals at risk should be repositioned as a response to skin inspection and according to individual need (Rycroft-Malone, 2000). They tend to agree (quite strongly) that this should not be ritualistic. In other words, routine care should not mean ritualized care, but should be individualized.

Routine turning or following a turning schedule (Lowthian, 1979) in itself may not be harmful and could have positive benefits. For instance, Norton (1975) implies that intensive nursing input is necessary to ensure frequent turns to prevent pressure ulcers. She comments that there was a reduction of incidence of pressure ulcers (from 24% to 9%) when patients with a Norton risk score of less than fourteen were 'intensively nursed', ie. mainly two-hourly turns recorded on a 'position time rota'.

The notion of two-hourly intervals has become a matter of custom and practice in some establishments. Anecdotally, it has been attributed to the length of time it took for nurses in the Crimean War hospitals to work their way down one side of a ward and up the other. A more contemporary origin could have been the spinal unit overseen by Sir Ludwig Guttman (Guttman, 1953, 1973). He introduced half-hourly to three-hourly turning for his spinal patients. Similarly, it is alluded to by Gardner and Anderson (1948), who utilized alternating pressure mattresses to save nursing time, thereby reducing the need for such frequent turning.

Unfortunately, turning regimens can impose big demands on nurses, and it is sometimes claimed that because of staff shortage, they do not have enough time to devote to turning (McDougall, 1976; Exton-Smith, 1987; Bliss, 1990; Hawkins *et al*, 1999).

A study in the United States (Helme, 1994) aimed to assess whether carers in long-term care facilities knew how often residents needed to be repositioned, ie. the recommendations of the US guidelines (Agency for Health Care Policy and Research, 1992). The researchers in this study also wanted to find out what interfered with nursing compliance and a unit's policy on turning. The results were analysed with reference to a convenience sample comprised of nursing assistants (people who had six weeks of classroom training and clinical experience, $n = 198$), registered and licensed practical nurses (the latter are akin to state-enrolled nurses, $n = 86$) and supervisory nurses ($n = 40$). The overall response rate to the questionnaires was 87%.

All groups agreed overwhelmingly that two-hour turn intervals were needed, and the majority agreed that they used a turn schedule (a turning clock chart usually displayed near the bed). A variety of mechanisms was said to have been used to reinforce practice, including intercom announcements, according to twenty-three respondents (8%). Interestingly, 166 (62%) of the bedside care givers said that responsibility for ensuring turns fell to their supervisors, and only eighty-two (29%) thought it was their own responsibility. Indeed, the supervisors acknowledged that compliance with the turning policy decreased when it was not reinforced by inspection rounds.

A study by Knox *et al* (1994) tried to validate the use of two-hourly turns relative to the effects of one- and one-and-a-half-hourly turns and to evaluate whether this affected interface pressures, skin temperature and skin colour changes. There were some conceptual difficulties with this research, eg. that interface pressure at the start and finish of a period in a given posture reflected internal capillary pressure. Nevertheless, the study demonstrated that even in rigorously controlled circumstances, observers can have little confidence in what they see on the skin surface. On the other methodological extreme (namely to measure one thing and assume it is directly related to another), Keane (1978), basing his calculations on studies of sleep, stated that one gross postural change would be required every 11.6 minutes to prevent pressure ulcers. He further advocated turns to a maximum of 124° in 4.5 minutes to provide a large safe margin for the prevention of pressure ulcers.

A pressure-relieving technique called the 30° tilt, described by Preston (1984), does not necessitate turning patients completely onto their side. It is achieved by placing ordinary pillows so that the trochanters are raised to create an angle of 30° between the supine patient and the bed. The trochanters and sacrum are virtually free of direct pressure in that position. The efficacy of the technique has been evaluated in terms of skin oxygen tension, on the premise that a reduction of the latter is an indicator of likely pressure damage (Seiler *et al*, 1983, 1986). In the two studies combined, a total of fifteen healthy women and six healthy men was used to test the differences between skin oxygen tension (SOT) while lying in various positions. The control position was prone, ie. no pressure on the trochanters or sacrum. This was compared with supine, on the side or at 30° tilt.

There were no significant differences between SOTs in the prone position and the unloaded (side or 30° tilt) positions, but the supine position showed a significant reduction in SOT over the prone position ($P<0.005$ on a standard mattress and $P<0.05$ on a 'supersoft' mattress). Although the study was not performed on large numbers and did not involve elderly patients at real risk of pressure damage, Seiler *et al* (1986) claimed to have seen a consistent drop in the prevalence of pressure ulcers in their hospital over the five years in which they had used the technique.

Despite the absence of clinical trials, the tilt may be a useful and well tolerated method of reducing risk, although the period to advocate between repositioning may be as low as hourly (Clark, 1998). There are some data (from healthy volunteers) to support the belief that oxygen impairment to the skin is worse in the 90° lateral position than when tilted to 30° (Colin *et al*, 1996). However, there has been debate as to the efficacy of the 30° tilt (Gebhardt, 2000, 2001; Hampton, 2001a). The arguments focus on whether the patient can be properly maintained with the legs at 180° to the trunk, that being (supposedly) the best position to ensure relief of pressure from the bony prominences (Hampton, 2001b). Gebhardt (2000) rightly cautions against assuming that it is a universally useful technique, citing a Japanese trial (Sanada, 2000) that showed a 100% increase in incidence of pressure ulceration after the method had been introduced.

Necessary turns or not

What happens if there are no other means of relieving pressure than to turn patients, as is the case in some parts of the world and even in this country? Although some staff might assume that patients do not need turning while on alternating-pressure air mattresses (APAMs), no systematic research can be found to quantify the assertion. In fact, there are reasons why turning, quite apart from the relief of pressure, may be considered helpful and necessary (Hawkins *et al*, 1999). These are issues ranging from maintaining musculoskeletal function to psychosocial stimulation.

Perhaps a rule of thumb would be that a planned period of skin observation should start with hourly inspection in the acutely ill, ie. when they are turned. The interval could be increased when one is convinced that erythema has resolved over the bony prominences after half an hour of complete relief. This would be done for all patients thought to be at risk of pressure ulceration, even while on high-tech pressure-reducing equipment. A chart (Lowthian, 1979) would aid communication of what position a patient is meant to be in at a given time.

Risk assessment and choices

Associating risk assessment with choices of equipment is fraught with danger because most, if not all, types of equipment have never been tested to justify whether this is statistically warranted (Maylor and Roberts, 1999; Maylor, 2001a; Stanton, 2001). However, in the majority of cases, nurses do know how to recognize a patient at risk of pressure damage (Hergenroeder *et al*, 1992); they know what equipment to recommend for them (Halfens and Eggink, 1995; Maylor and Torrance, 1999a), and they tend to be overcautious (opting for more sophisticated levels of prevention than strictly necessary; Maylor, 1999).

Also, the argument that there is not enough equipment to provide for patients was not supported over several years of prevalence studies (Torrance and Maylor, 1999). This reinforces the suspicion that nurses are reactive rather than proactive (Gunningberg *et al*, 2000). In short, choices of pressure-reducing equipment and techniques need to be tailored to the individual. Moreover, it can be argued that speed of access to pressure reduction during an acute phase of illness (a marker of which is incontinence), when patients cannot lift themselves, is more important than trying to make unwarranted comparisons between equipment relative to notional risk levels (Maylor, 2001a).

With no visible evidence of pressure damage, nurses may be less likely to argue for provisional investment in apparatus, simply because they cannot prove that a pressure ulcer would have occurred if they had not prevented it. The personal control expectancies of care staff have been shown to have important associations with departmental prevalence of ulcers (Maylor and Torrance, 1999b; Maylor, 2000). Paradoxically, the more sisters believe that they personally control pressure ulcer prevention, the higher the departmental prevalence; the more they think pressure ulcer prevention cannot be controlled, the lower the prevalence (Maylor, 1999). An explanation of this paradox is that the more controlling types of sisters set other priorities for staff at the expense of pressure ulcer prevention, while the fatalistic types, in some way, intervene to stave off what they imagine to be inevitable.

Nursing home staff may not react in the same way as hospital counterparts, although this has not yet been tested. But it could be argued that in hospital, sisters have to juggle many priorities, whereas a patient sent to a nursing home with a pressure ulcer becomes a particular focus of attention.

Residents discharged from hospital with pressure ulcers

The majority of pressure damage occurs in the first few days after admission with an acute episode of illness (Versluysen, 1985, 1986; Hawthorn and Nyquist, 1988; Gebhardt, 1992; Torrance and Maylor, 1999). Furthermore, studies consistently show that community settings, as opposed to hospitals, generally have lower prevalence of pressure ulcers (Oot-Giromini, 1993; Meehan, 1994; Thoroddsen, 1999).

United Kingdom data concerning the numbers of pressure ulcers in nursing and residential homes are rarely published, and although there are papers from abroad, the term 'nursing home' may be misleading, as some of these institutions, for example in Holland, can be likened to NHS intermediate care facilities. It seems fair to conclude that residents are more likely to be discharged with a pressure ulcer than to be sent into hospital with one. If true, it inevitably gives rise to difficulties for nursing and residential homes, because it means accepting transferred responsibility for the consequences of damage, although not of the original cause.

Along with this comes the inherited problem of providing adequate care in order to prevent deterioration and to encourage healing. The cost in human and financial terms is 'inherited' by patients and carers outside the acute setting. On the other hand, problems occur for a hospital in that it wants to discharge patients as soon as possible because there is demand for rapid throughput. Some blame delay of discharge on lack of equipment in the nursing and residential home, although miracles do occur and a 'patient' in need of an APAM on Thursday becomes a 'resident' who can take up a bed and walk on Friday.

From the nursing and residential home's point of view, should they provide a directly equivalent APAM to the one the resident had in hospital? The first principle would be to judge whether the resident must be treated in the same way in both settings. Logic dictates that there should be initial agreement on the likely level of pressure reduction with staff in the hospital, particularly if a method of risk assessment or a policy or guideline is used locally. If the resident has no ulcer, the best equipment and interventions available will afford some protection for the residents until such time as their true status can be gauged in their home environment. 'Stepping down', ie. using progressively less costly or sophisticated techniques, could follow the pattern suggested above in relation to recognition of safe intervals to allow for erythema to disappear.

'Normal beds'

The vast majority of people in the West sleep on some sort of static bed frame with a sprung mattress, and these divan-type beds are still seen in mental health, nursing home and residential care settings. To date, many questions remain unanswered about how 'normal' beds affect patient care. For example, does a mattress become conformed to the shape of its owner to the extent that frequent use increases the surface area of the body in contact with it (thereby reducing point pressure)? If this is true, when admitted to hospital in a physiologically vulnerable state, do other parts of the body unaccustomed to bearing weight suffer detrimentally from the new and higher levels of point pressure? Would it be less harmful to send the patients to hospital on their own bed? These are conjectural but possibly important research questions.

Comfort might be harmful

It is likely that people equate softness with comfort (and with lower potential for pressure damage). But this is too simplistic and could lull staff into a false sense of security, if only for the fact that patients have different views on what constitutes comfort (Hampton, 1999).

An Indian paper (Koul *et al*, 2000) described the association between new back pain and sleeping on a foam mattress in hospital rather than the usual cotton mattress; once back at home, the pain disappeared. So the firmer mattresses was more suitable (to the extent that some patients defaulted on appointments because of discomfort from the hospital mattresses).

This contrasted with significant reduction in pain and increased quality of sleep in a USA study of the use of an inflatable air mattress rather than the patient's own 'innerspring' mattress (Monsein *et al*, 2000). However, a German study (Knobel, 1996) serves as another warning that soft is not always best. Knobel used a video camera to track patient activities in a nursing home context after the patients had slept on a 'supersoft' mattress rather than a conventional hospital mattress. His pilot study found that soft mattresses could restrict mobility, reduce orientation and impair human function, particularly perception.

A Swedish study of sleep quality and comfort illustrated two factors: first, that some prefer hard rather than soft mattresses and vice versa, and second, that reported sleep quality is not necessarily reflected in the measured sleep data (Bader and Engdal, 2000). In other words, people say they slept badly but exhibited less outward signs of this and vice versa.

Integrating the above observations, it appears that softness or hardness of a mattress is experienced in different ways, with effects varying from backache to disorientation and reduced mobility. If the sleep patterns are construed by an observer as signifying 'good' depth of sleep but by the sleeper as 'bad', this might indicate that softer mattresses are inhibiting sleep mobility, with detrimental consequences in terms of pressure ulcer development (Barbenel *et al*, 1986). Thus, mattresses softer than the patients' norm might cause them problems.

This possibility is strengthened by results from a study in the USA. Here, observations of palliative patients cared for at home showed that new pressure ulcers were detected in 67% of patients on 'convoluted foam' mattresses and in 18% on their own mattress (significant with an *2 test, but probability level unreported) (Stoneberg *et al*, 1986).

All in all, care has to be taken to select a mattress that the patients can tolerate, that promotes their comfort (as subjectively reported by them) but that leaves no persistent erythema on bony prominences (Agency for Health Care Policy and Research, 1992; Rycroft-Malone, 2000). It may be that 'sinking in' to a soft mattress or overlay counteracts the residual strength of older, poorly or disabled people that they have hitherto used to make macro- or micro-movements to protect themselves from the ischaemic effects of pressure.

Conclusions

This chapter has attempted to review evidence regarding the efficacy of pressure-reducing equipment and techniques. The number of trials and evaluations where statistics and data are analysed is small, but a pattern and several themes have emerged. The pattern is one of consistent benefit derived from alternating pressure. It can be achieved by electro-mechanical means or by manual repositioning.

Because of the ethical desire to prevent harm to patients, it has not been possible directly to compare the less costly APAMs with those that are much more expensive. But there have been recent challenges to the use of APAMs, namely by static air-filled, fluid-filled or viscoelastic thermal reactive foams. At least two implications follow; first, patients are physiologically protected not by keeping points of pressure intermittently low, but by the fact that metabolic processes are not disrupted by periods of higher pressure spread across various body sites on the better APAMs, and second, continuous static pressure surfaces may be appearing that match the performance of APAMs for the majority of patients. In the first situation, ie. APAMs, the mattress moves, but in the second situation, ie. static surfaces, the patient moves. As long as either moves sufficiently, the constant challenges to cell perfusion never go beyond the point of no return (localized thrombosis).

The nursing skill is to judge whether a piece of equipment is 'up to the job' for an individual or whether additional or alternative methods need to be implemented.

How can the nurse and patient decide what is suitable? Probably not by recourse to notional specifications tying risk assessment scores with an assumed hierarchy of equipment. Observation of the tissue response to relief of pressure is a key skill. The intention should surely be to provide the best method (particularly when people are acutely ill and cannot move themselves off a bed or chair) and then to carefully 'step down' as a controlled response to resolving erythema on vulnerable prominences. That would be time and money well spent, not least because resources would not be in use for longer than they need to be, and it should encourage a philosophy of recovery, not dependency.

Key points

⌘ Changing an individual's position is perhaps the simplest tactic that ......
    the duration of prolonged loading on the skin's soft tissues.

⌘ There remains considerable confusion regarding this apparently simple
    intervention with uncertainty over the frequency of repositioning, the
    positions adopted following repositioning and the effect of repositioning on
    pressure ulcer development.

⌘ There remains a clear need for further research into the effectiveness and
    efficiency of the manual reposition of patients to avoid pressure ulcer
    development.

References

Agency for Health Care Policy and Research (1992) *Clinical Practice Guideline Number 3: Pressure Ulcers in Adults: Prediction and Prevention*. US Department of Health and Human Sciences, Rockville, Maryland

Agency for Heath Care Policy and Research (1994 [reviewed 2000]) *Clinical Practice Guideline Number 15. Treatment of Pressure Ulcers*. US Department of Health and Human Services, Rockville, Maryland

Bader G, Engdal S (2000) The influence of bed firmness on sleep quality. *Appl Ergon* **31**(5): 487–97

Barbenel J, Ferguson-Pell M, Kennedy R (1986) Mobility of elderly patients in bed. *J Am Geriatr Soc* **34**: 633–6

Bliss M (1990) Geriatric Medicine. In: Bader DL, ed. *Pressure Sores: Clinical Practice and Scientific Approach*. Macmillan Press, Basingstoke: 65–80

Clark M (1998) Repositioning to prevent pressure sores — what is the evidence? *Nurs Stand* **13**(3): 58–64

Colin D, Abraham P, Preault L *et al* (1996) Comparison of 90° and 30° laterally inclined positions in the prevention of pressure ulcers using transcutaneous oxygen and carbon dioxide pressures. *Adv Wound Care* **9**(3): 35–8

Exton-Smith N (1987) The patient's not for turning. *Nurs Times* **83**(42): 42–4

Gardner J, Anderson R (1948) Alternating pressure alleviates bedsores. *Modern Hospital* **71**: 72–3

Gebhardt K (1992) Preventing pressure sores in orthopaedics. *Nurs Stand* **6**(23 Suppl): 4–6

Gebhardt K (2000) Editorial. New rituals for old. *J Tissue Viability* **10**(4): 131–2

Gebhardt K (2001) Appropriate use of the 30-degree tilt. *Br J Nurs* **10**(11 Suppl): 8

Gunningberg L, Lindholm C, Carlsson M *et al* (2000) The development of pressure ulcers in patients with hip fractures: inadequate nursing documentation is still a problem. *J Adv Nurs* **31**(5): 1155–64

Guttman L (1953) The treatment and rehabilitation of patients with injuries of the spinal cord. In: Cope Z, ed. *Medical History of the Second World War, Surgery*. HMSO, London: 422–516

Guttman L (1973) *Spinal Cord Injuries: Comprehensive Management and Research*. Blackwell Scientific, Oxford

Halfens R, Eggink M (1995) Knowledge, beliefs and use of nursing methods in preventing pressure sore in Dutch hospitals. *Int J Nurs Stud* **32**(1): 16–26

Hampton S (1999) Efficacy and cost-effectiveness of the Thermo contour mattress. *Br J Nurs* **8**(15): 990–6

Hampton S (2001a) Pressure ulcer care: can we learn from poorer countries? *Br J Nurs* **10**(6 Suppl): 4

Hampton S (2001b) Should we use the 30-degree tilt? *J Wound Care* **10**(8): 344

Hawkins S, Stone K, Plummer L (1999) An holistic approach to turning patients. *Nurs Stand* **14**(3): 52–6

Hawthorn P, Nyquist R (1988) The incidence of pressure sores amongst a group of elderly patients with fractured neck of femur. *Care - Sci Pract* **6**(1): 3–7

Helme T (1994) Position changes for residents in long-term care. *Adv Wound Care* **7**(5): 57–61

Hergenroeder P, Mosher C, Sebo D (1992) Pressure ulcer assessment — simple or complex? *Decubitus* **5**(14): 42–7

Kanj L, Wilking SVB, Phillips T (1998) Pressure ulcers. *J Am Acad Dermatol* **38**(4): 517–38

Keane F (1978) The minimum physiological mobility requirement for man supported on a soft surface. *Paraplegia* **16**: 383–9

Knobel S (1996) Getting up on the right side of the bed ... the influence of supersoft mattresses on the mobility of elderly nursing home patients. *Pflege* **9**(2): 134–9

Knox D, Anderson T, Anderson P (1994) Effects of different turn intervals on skin of healthy older adults. *Adv Wound Care* **7**(1): 48–56

Koul P, Bhat M, Lone A *et al* (2000) The foam mattress-back syndrome. *J Assoc Physicians India* **48**(9): 901–2

Lowthian P (1979) Turning clock system to prevent pressure sores. *Nurs Mirror* **148**(21): 30–1

Maylor, M (1999) Controlling the pressure: an investigation of knowledge, locus of control, and value of pressure sore prevention in relation to prevalence. Unpublished PhD. University of Glamorgan, Glamorgan

Maylor M (2000) Investigating the value of pressure sore prevention. *Br J Nurs* **9**(12 Suppl): 50–1

Maylor M (2001a). Pressure reducing equipment 1: general testing issues. *Nurs Residential Care* **3**(9): 426–33

Maylor M (2001b) Debating the relative unimportance of pressure reducing equipment. *Br J Nurs* **10**(15): 1162–5

Maylor M, Roberts A (1999) A comparison of three risk assessment scales. *Prof Nurse* **14**(9): 629–32

Maylor M, Torrance C (1999a) Pressure sore survey part 2: nurses' knowledge. *J Wound Care* **8**(2): 49–52

Maylor M, Torrance C (1999b) Pressure sore survey part 3: locus of control. *J Wound Care* **8**(3): 101–5

McDougall A (1976) Clinical aspects of bed sore prevention and treatment. In: Kenedi R, Cowden J, Scales J, eds. *Bed Sore Biomechanics*. MacMillan, London and Basingstoke: 161–7

Meehan M (1994) National Pressure Ulcer Prevalence Survey. *Adv Wound Care* **7**(3): 27–38

Monsein M, Corbin T, Culliton P *et al* (2000) Short-term outcomes of chronic back pain patients on an airbed *vs* innerspring mattresses. Online at: http://www.medscape.com/Medscape/GeneralMedicine/journal/2000/v02.n05/mgm0911.corb/432585.html (accessed 12 November 2001)

Norton D (1975) Research and the problem of pressure sores. *Nurs Mirror* **14**: 65–8

Oot-Giromini B (1993) Pressure ulcer prevalence, incidence and associated risk factors in the community. *Decubitus* **6**(5): 24–32

Preston K (1984) Positioning for comfort and pressure relief: the 30 degree alternative. *Care Sci Pract* **6**(4): 116–19

Rycroft-Malone J (2000) *Clinical Practice Guidelines. Pressure Ulcer Risk Assessment and Prevention*. Royal College of Nursing, London

Sanada H (2000) Current issues in pressure ulcer management of the bedfast elderly in Japan. In: Oita Medical University, ed. Rehabilitation Society of Japan, Special Interest Group, Prevention and Management of Pressure Sores. International Symposium on Pressure Sore Prevention in 2000 — Scientific Challenge Toward Pressure Sore 'Zero' Incidence. Oita: the Society and the University: 65–73

Seiler W, Allen S, Stahelin H (1983) Decubitus ulcer prevention: a new investigative method using transcutaneous oxygen tension measurement. *J Am Geriatr Soc* **31**(12): 786–9

Seiler W, Allen S, Stahelin H (1986) Influence of the 30° laterally inclined position and the 'Super-soft' 3-piece mattress on skin oxygen tension on areas of maximum pressure — implications for pressure sore prevention. *Gerontology* **32**: 158–66

Stanton J (2001) A nurse's aid to clinical selection of pressure-reducing equipment. *Br J Nurs* **10**(15 Suppl): 16–28

Stoneberg C, Pitcock N, Myton C (1986) Pressure sores in the homebound: one solution. *Am J Nurs* **86**(4): 426–8

Thoroddsen A (1999) Pressure sore prevalence: a national survey. *J Clin Nurs* **8**(2): 170–9

Torrance C, Maylor M (1999) Pressure sore survey: part one. *J Wound Care* **8**(1): 27–30

Versluysen M (1985) Pressure sores in elderly patients. The epidemiology related to hip operations. *J Bone Joint Surg* **67**(1): 10–13

Versluysen M (1986) How elderly patients develop pressure ulcers in hospital. *Br Med J* **292**: 1311–13

7

Evaluation of alternating-pressure air mattresses: How to do it

Shyam VS Rithalia

Although many different type of alternating-pressure air mattresses (APAMs) are used for the prevention and treatment of pressure ulcers, few high quality randomised controlled trials (RCTs) are available on which to base purchasing decisions. Faced with this situation, physiological measurements are increasingly being used as a surrogate. Laboratory evaluation techniques have centered largely on interface pressure (IP) measurement, typically analysing discrete maximum and minimum levels, or average pressure. However, since pressure relief is time varying, a time-based analysis technique is more suitable for performance assessment. Measurements of IP, mattress air-cells pressure (AP), skin tissue perfusion using laser Doppler (LD) fluxmetry and transcutaneous oxygen (tcPO$_2$) and carbon dioxide (tcPCO$_2$) were taken simultaneously over at least two alternating cycles. Duration of IP below three thresholds (30, 20, and 10 mm Hg), as well as area under the tcPO$_2$, tcPCO$_2$ and LD curves were calculated automatically using a computerised rig. Ten healthy volunteers were used to evaluate the pressure relieving characteristics of two different designs of APAMs. Results indicated significant differences between the products. During deflation phase of the cycle contact pressures on the heel were significantly lower (p<0.0001) on the device whose inflation pressure was significantly higher, although there was no significant difference in deflation pressure. Therefore, it is important to note that low air cell pressures do not necessarily produce lower IPs under the heel, contrary to the intuitive classical notion. These techniques could assist in the selection of alternating or dynamic surfaces of any description with further clinical validation.

Introduction

Pressure ulcers cause great pain and suffering to patients. They also impose unnecessary psychological and physical strain on the dedicated nursing staff and carers. Their treatment is both costly and time consuming (Tingle, 1998; Hibbs, 1988; Robertson, 1987). Prevention of pressure sores is important, as they are often preventable. This will reduce unnecessary expenditure to the National Health Service (NHS) and unnecessary misery to the patient. Frequent, two-hourly round the clock, turning of patients is a time honoured and proven method of pressure ulcer prevention (Panel for the Prediction and Prevention of Pressure Ulcers in Adults, 1992; Guttmann, 1976). However, manual turning is labour intensive and may also induce pain in some patients (Exton-Smith, 1987; Green, 1976). Other effective ways of reducing the detrimental effects of external pressure include the use of devices (Fletcher, 1993; Redfern, 1973) which redistribute body weight more evenly (pressure-reducing or static surfaces) and devices (Dunford,

1991; Bedford *et al*, 1961) which cyclically change the area of exposure to pressure (pressure-relieving or alternating surfaces). Pressure relief (PR) is defined as the ability of a support surface to substantially remove localised pressure.

Alternating surfaces are amongst the most popular devices for the prevention and treatment of pressure ulcers (Anon, 1996; Bliss and Thomas, 1993; Willis 1996). In recent years, many new APAMs have become commercially available. They vary considerably in their design, cost, reliability, maintenance and ease of use (Rithalia, 1995; Lockyer-Stevens, 1994). These devices appear to offer the benefit of actively encouraging tissue perfusion by alternately increasing and decreasing the pressure exerted under the body by the supporting surface. Their effectiveness can only be definitively determined by large scale controlled clinical trials which are difficult to organise, analyse and fund (Bliss, 1993). There is also a great deal of interest in finding other ways of assessing the possible efficacy of different types of support surfaces (Mcleod, 1997; Rithalia, 1991).

The most commonly quoted method, both by researchers and commercial vendors of support surfaces, has been the measurement of interface pressure (IP). This is usually done by placing a pressure transducer between the body and the support surface (Pring and Millman, 1998; Berijan *et al*, 1983; Grant, 1981). The discrete measurements of maximum, minimum and mean or average IP at specific bony prominences, such as the sacrum, trochanter and the heel have been the most commonly used parameters (Sideranko *et al*, 1992; Maklebust *et al*, 1986). These measurements give no indication of the time during which low IP is experienced. It would be more useful to be able to measure pressure relief index (PRI). PRI is defined as the proportion of the time-cycle of the device during which the IP is below a certain limit (Mcleod, 1997). The higher the proportion, the more likely it is to be of benefit. It is, however, important to remember that a single method of assessment may not result in providing appropriate information (Price *et al*, 1999). There has also been a growing interest, in recent years, in the assessment of skin tissue perfusion (Xakellios *et al*, 1991; Wyss *et al*, 1988; McCollumn *et al*, 1986) by measurement of transcutaneous oxygen ($tcPO_2$) and carbon dioxide ($tcPCO_2$). Several investigators have used $tcPO_2$ and $tcPCO_2$ monitoring to compare support surfaces (Colin *et al*, 1996; Salisbury, 1985). These assessed skin tissue perfusion under the sacrum of subjects lying supine on a mattress. Recently, the effect of pressure-relief on heel blood flow has also been investigated using laser Doppler (LD) monitor (Rithalia and Russell, 2003; Mayrovitz and Smith, 1998)

At Salford, a computerised system (*Figure 7.1*) has been developed which measures interface pressure (IP), air cell pressure (AP) and skin tissue perfusion using transcutaneous gases or laser Doppler flowmetry. A graphical programming language (Lab View, National Instruments Inc, USA) was used to develop the monitoring system. The system calculates pressure-time characteristics (Rithalia and Gonsalkorale, 1998) and more recently analysis of perfusion time-integral data has also been added (Rithalia and Russell, 2003; Rithalia and Gonsalkorale, 2000). The simultaneous monitoring of these parameters in the evaluation of time-varying support surfaces is fairly new and hence novel techniques are required to interpret the data. The present study illustrates the approach taken to the analysis of continuous measurements and, as an example, two different approaches to the design of APAMs, low AP (Duo, Hill-Rom Ltd, UK) and high AP (Nimbus 3, Huntleigh Healthcare Ltd, UK) were investigated using PRI and blood perfusion measurements.

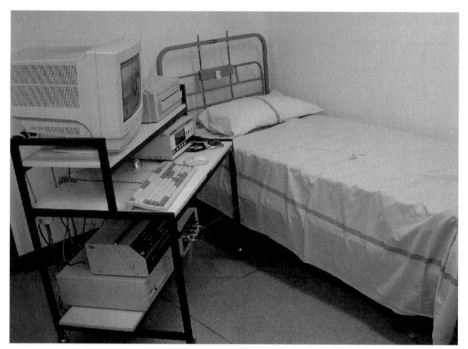

Figure 7.1: The Nimbus 3 replacement mattress connected to the computerised system

Methods and materials

For each product the following measurements and data were acquired:

- mean maximum and minimum interface pressures
- mean peak air pressures in the mattresses
- interface pressure durations below 30, 20 and 10 mm Hg over a sixty-minute period
- mean maximum $tcPCO_2$ and minimum $tcPO_2$
- mean area under the $tcPO_2$ and $tcPCO_2$ curves
- mean maximum LD blood perfusion
- mean area under LD blood perfusion curves
- comments regarding perceived comfort level
- operational reliability and general ease of use.

Subjects

A total of ten healthy subjects participated in the investigation for interface pressure and skin tissue perfusion measurements. They were recruited from postgraduate students and staff of the University of Salford. Their ages, weights and heights ranged from twenty-two to sixty-two (mean ± SD, 35.8 ± 12.7) years, 56 to 95 (71.5 ± 11.1) kg and 1.60 to 1.91(1.70 ± 0.10) m respectively. All subjects were identified as being healthy and had the procedure fully explained to them. Their written consent was obtained prior to the commencement of the measurements. Subjects were chosen not completely at random, but rather to provide a spread of males and females with a reasonable range of weights, heights and ages.

Procedure

Mattress systems were switched on and allowed to operate for at least thirty minutes prior to testing. Whilst the mattress was inflating, the subjects were weighed, their heights recorded and they were asked their age. A standard hospital sheet was placed on the mattress. The subjects were asked to lie on the bed, whilst wearing normal light clothing, with legs uncrossed and arms at the sides. They were allowed to position themselves so that they were comfortable using two standard pillows to support their head. Room temperature was regulated between 23 and 26°C during all measurements.

The anatomical position of body was determined by palpation and a single pneumatic transducer (OPM, model II, Talley Group Ltd, UK) placed between the site of measurement and the support surface. Measurements of interface pressure were carried out continuously under the sacrum and heel in the supine position, left trochanter in the side-lying position, and buttock in the sitting position with bed back rest at forty-five degrees. Care was used to avoid creases in clothing or the bed sheet and that the transducer did not lie over a seam in any clothing. The transducer was placed on the centre of a cell so that it did not fall into gaps between inflating and deflating cells. It was decided that this was best done by initially placing the transducer on an inflated cell to minimise the possibility of it moving and that it could be certain that it was centred over the mattress cell.

Measurements of the $tcPO_2$ and $tcPCO_2$ (TCM3, Radiometer A/S, Denmark) were made simultaneously with interface pressure on the sacrum. The skin at the electrode application site was first degreased with alcohol, then cleansed and dried. The electrode was applied to the skin by means of double-sided adhesive rings. The temperature of the $tcPO_2/tcPCO_2$ sensor was set at 44°C during calibration and for all measurements. Once the sensor was attached a period of twenty to thirty minutes was allowed for stabilisation of the recordings and base-line readings were taken while the subject side-lying on the left trochanter. The subject was then positioned carefully in such a way that the sensors rested on the top of an inflated cell of the mattress. Pressure concentration on the sensors attached to the sacrum, while lying supine, was diffused by covering the electrode with therapeutic putty. After the skin gas measurements, a further five- to ten-minute period was allowed before the sensors removed and their calibration rechecked.

For simultaneous measurements of LD blood flow and IP on the heel, the subjects were asked to lie supine on the bed. Care was taken to place both left and right heels on the centre of the same air cell of the mattress. Interface pressure transducer was placed under the right heel and laser Doppler probe (Softflo, model BPM2, Vasamedics Inc, USA) on the left heel with the feet in a neutral position in order to maintain uniformity of the method throughout the study.

All measurements were taken over at least two alternating cycles. Statistical analysis was performed by using a computer programme (Analyse-It, Analyse-It Software Ltd, Leeds, UK). Differences between various pressures and blood perfusion values over one cycle were analysed using Student's t-test or the Wilcoxon's matched-pairs signed-rank test depending on whether or not data were normally distributed. A difference was considered significant when $p<0.05$.

The subjects were asked regarding comfort or discomfort such as, hardness of the surface, stickiness, roughness, itching or irritation, and which of the two surfaces they found most comfortable. During the trial period of approximately three months on the ward, assessments were made by the nursing staff of factors such as stability of the patients on the APAMs, durability, cleaning, ease of use and user's acceptability.

Description and results

A brief description of each APAM with its principles of operation is presented. Initially, the results obtained were in the form of pressure/time graph output with transcutaneous gas tracing (*Figure 7.2*) and LD blood perfusion curve (*Figure 7.3*). Skin tissue perfusion is expressed as the area under the $tcPO_2$, $tcPCO_2$ (*Table 7.1*) and LD curves (*Table 7.2*) in arbitrary units. Finally they are presented numerically as bar charts with mean ± standard deviation (*Figures 7.4–6*). The pressure relieving (PR) characteristics of the mattresses are presented in terms of IP, $tcPO_2$, $tcPCO_2$ and LD values. All data are analysed over a period of one complete cycle.

Table 7.1: Summary of IP, AP, PRI and perfusion values under the heel

	Duo			Nimbus 3			
Observations	Mean	± SD	Range	Mean	± SD	Range	*P* values
Maximum IP (mmHg)	150	31	108–196	134	23	100–187	0.189
Minimum IP (mmHg)	69	19	37–98	20	5	13–30	<0.001*
Peak air pressure (mmHg)	7	1	6–8	32	4	29–42	<0.002*
Perfusion starts @ IP (mmHg)	83	14	68110	62	9	48–75	<0.002*
Peak perfusion (AU)	15	5	4–21	68	32	35–115	<0.01*
Perfusion/cycle (AU)	3511	1173	2059–5289	12022	6538	2237–17151	<0.002*
PRI <30 mmHg (min/hour)	0	0	0	15	4	0–22	–
PRI <20 mmHg (min/hour)	0	0	0	7	5	0–14	–

* statistically significant difference at *p*<0.05

Table 7.2: Details of PRI, $tcPO_2$ and $tcPCO_2$ under the sacrum

	Duo			Nimbus 3			
Observations	Mean	± SD	Range	Mean	± SD	Range	*P* values
Base-line TcPO$_2$ (mmHg)	89.2	6.4	76–96	89.1	6.8	76–96	0.832
Base-line tcPCO$_2$ (mmHg)	39.7	2.8	33–42	39.9	2.8	33–43	0.5000
Lowest tcPO$_2$ (mmHg)	73.3	5.0	67–81	62.9	10.6	43–76	0.0154*
Highest tcPCO$_2$ (mmHg)	44.7	4.4	36–51	44.3	3.8	35–48	1.0000
Area under tcPO$_2$ curve (AU)	7764.5	3720.1	2250–13760	9627.9	3038.7	5492–13759	0.2271
Area under tcPCO2 curve (AU)	2250.3	1750.3	182–4860	1228.8	725.5	359–2644	0.0727
PRI <30 mmHg (min/hour)	59.7	0.9	57–60	47.3	9.4	34.60	0.0078*
PRI <20 mmHg (min/hour)	48.1	21.3	2–80	34.6	5.1	29–46	0.1055
PRI <10 mmHg (min/hour)	10.0	16.4	0–49	18.4	8.9	0–29	0.2500

* statistically significant difference at *p*<0.05

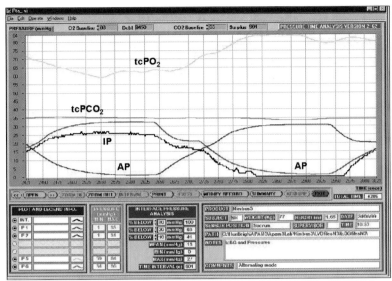

Figure 7.2: A typical graph showing interface pressure (IP), air cell pressures (AP), transcutaneous oxygen (tcPO$_2$) and carbon dioxide (tcPCO$_2$) at the sacrum

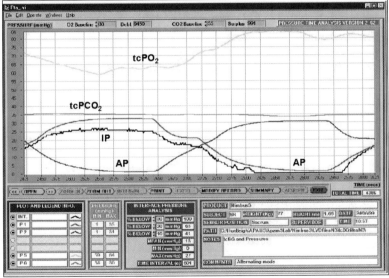

Figure 7.3: A typical graph showing interface pressure (IP), air cell pressures (AP), and laser Doppler trace on heel

Low AP (Duo) mattress

The Duo™ system consists of two very complex and independent elements: a mattress with 19 air cell enclosed in a cover and a De.teq™ pressure control module. The mattress incorporates a low air pressure heel zone (Real Heel™) at the foot end, which operates in both continuous and alternating therapy modes. The lower heel zone operates at five minutes cycle time, while the upper torso section has a cycle time of ten minutes. The De.teq™ pressure control module ensures that all the air cells are automatically regulated at the lowest possible support pressure. All of these functions, including CPR mode, are controlled by a compact, lightweight and easy to use control pendant. However, the mattress system is heavy and cumbersome to move from one bed frame to another.

For the ten subjects, the overall maximum interface pressure values during inflation phase of the cycle under the heel were 149.6 ± 30.6 mmHg and during deflation phase the minimum values were 69.4 ± 18.8 mmHg. The mean maximum air cell pressure values for the heel were 7.2 ± 0.6 mmHg. Interface pressures at the heel remained above 30 mm Hg during the whole cycle for all subjects. In comparison with the Nimbus 3 (air cell pressure = 31.6 ± 3.9 mm Hg), the Duo operated at significantly lower (p<0.0001) air cell inflation pressures for all measurements.

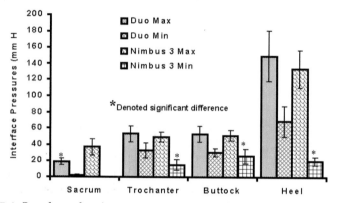

Figure 7.4: Bar chart showing mean maximum and minimum interface pressures at sacrum, trochanter, buttock and heel

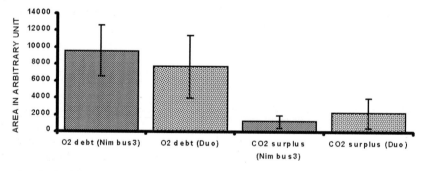

Figure 7.5: Bar chart showing tcPO$_2$ debt and tcPCO$_2$ surplus at the sacrum over a sixty-minute period

It was generally perceived as a comfortable mattress in supine position with pressure relieving characteristics (mean maximum IP= 19.8 ± 5.9 mmHg and PRI below 30 mmHg = 59.7 ± 0.9 min/h) at the sacrum better (p<0.0001) than the Nimbus 3 (mean maximum IP = 34.4 ± 6.0 mm Hg and PRI below 30 mm Hg = 47.3 ± 9.4 min/h). However, there was no significant difference in PRI below 20 mm Hg or carbon dioxide surplus values. Three out of ten subjects found Duo uncomfortable when used with an inclined backrest. Some of the subjects, especially the ones with low weight, tended to roll off the bed when side-lying during measurements at the trochanter.

High AP (Nimbus 3) mattress

This replacement mattress consists of twenty individual modular air cells having a figure-of-eight construction, placed transversely and connected alternately in two groups. One of the new developments is the inclusion of five Heelguard™ cells at the foot of the mattress. The lower foot cells have elastic bands with stiff plastic base, while fifteen upper cells are similar to foot cells but have no elastic loops. Each of the two groups is inflated and deflated with a cycle time of ten minutes. A sensor pad (Auto-matt™), which lies under the air cells, forms an integral part of pressure relief system. The Auto-matt™ can detect and automatically change the inflation pressure according to posture and subject weight. These aim to lower the peak interface pressure on soft tissue and generate greater levels of comfort.

For the ten subjects, the overall maximum interface pressure values during inflation phase of the cycle under the heel were 138.8 ± 20.1 mmHg and during deflation phase the minimum values were 19.6 ± 5.1 mm Hg. The time intervals calculated over sixty minutes when IP remained below arbitrarily chosen thresholds of 30 and 20 mmHg were 14.5 ± 6.9 (range $0 - 22$) and 3.8 ± 5.3 (range $0 - 14$) minutes respectively for the Nimbus. Skin LD levels integrated over time were significantly greater ($p<0.001$) for the Nimbus (12021.6 ± 6538.2 AU) compared with those for the Duo (3511.3 ± 1173.4 AU).

No significant differences in peak interface pressures were found between the two mattresses when they were used under the trochanter and buttock. But, Nimbus gave lower IPs during the deflation phase (trochanter, Duo = 32.8 ± 9.0 mmHg and Nimbus = 15.3 ± 6.5 mmHg; buttock, Duo = 30.4 ± 4.9 and Nimbus = 25.9 ± 9.0). There was a tendency for the cells to trap under one another in both mattresses when used in sitting position with bed headrest at an angle greater than 30 degrees. Two out of ten subjects reported discomfort due to the dragging action, or up and down motion, of the cells when Nimbus was used with an inclined backrest.

Discussion

APAMs work by a mechanism which pumps in air alternately in a given group of cells at a preset rate and time period to produce inflation of the cells. Then a mechanism operates to allow passive deflation of cells. Both the inflation pressure and time cycle is important for an optimum efficacy of the device (Gardner and Anderson, 1948; Dunford, 1991). For optimum comfort and pressure relief an APAM must be correctly inflated (Rithalia, 1995). The air pressure in the mattress should be directly proportional to the patient's weight, as well as surface area in contact with the mattress. High intermittent pressure may be more tolerable, using the criterion of histologically demonstrable tissue damage, than low constant pressure (Hussain, 1953). But high pressures, even for a short period of time, are uncomfortable (Trumble, 1930). Although both mattresses evaluated in this study were capable of relieving sacral interface pressures to below 10 mmHg, PRI values at these low pressures varied considerably. Therefore, caution should be used in making any conclusions based on a small number of subjects who may not represent a true spread of the general population.

A good correlation between arterial and cutaneous values has been shown by numerous investigators in patients with normal skin perfusion, but with impaired blood flow due to pressure on the electrode $tcPCO_2$ rises and $tcPO_2$ falls (Xakellis *et al*, 1991; Newson and Rolfe, 1982; Clutton-Brock and Rithalia, 1984). Therefore, together they form a fairly good monitoring system for assessing the adequacy of tissue oxygenation and carbon dioxide removal from the skin under pressure. With increasing pressure, a decrease in $tcPO_2$ and an increase in $tcPCO_2$ were seen, for example *Figure 7.3* in the present study. Although measurements are simple, reliable and sensitive to local variations in microcirculation, which exist in the skin under localised pressure, the size of the sensor is the main problem and false readings occur unless influence of direct pressure is diffused over a large area. Furthermore, since the transcutaneous electrodes need to be heated to 44°C, and the assessment lasted nearly three hours, this procedure caused discomfort even to the healthy subjects.

Both the Duo and Nimbus 3 varied peak inflation pressures according to posture and subject weight. Whilst this study identified significant differences in interface pressure relieving performance between the two products, the relationship between interface pressure measurement and clinical outcomes is as yet unclear. Ultimately, the effectiveness of these devices can only be fully demonstrated by controlled clinical trials (Bliss and Thomas, 1992). Meanwhile, based on current results, it appears that the Nimbus system has a theoretical advantage over the Duo in protecting skin tissue at the heel, trochanter and buttock from the deleterious effects of prolonged recumbency. It is interesting to note that the mattress that gave higher PRI values also showed greater tissue perfusion readings, thus indicating a direct positive relationship between PRI and skin tissue perfusion. From the combined results of IP and blood perfusion in healthy subjects, it seems that, to produce re-perfusion after loading an appropriate course of action is to provide periodic complete or near complete off-loading. In a recent study, using a cyclic pressure in a single air cell, Mayrovitz *et al* (2003) have also shown that complete heel-off-loading during a pressure-relief phase yielded a greater relative perfusion when compared with partial off-loading. Although the clinical evidence base is sparse, one clinical study (Russell and Reyholds, 2000) supports a relationship between PRI results (Rithalia and Health, 2000) and clinical outcome. It is also important to note that low air cell pressures do not necessarily produce lower IPs under the heel, contrary to the intuitive classical notion. One possible explanation for the apparent anomaly is that both the cell distribution and inter-cell pressure phase differences will have an effect on the way in which the body's weight is reacted through the support surface and hence on the interface pressure readings.

In summary, both the mattresses had certain limitations. The findings, however, should not be interpreted as the endorsement of one APAM or the criticism of the other mattress. The data were obtained objectively and it is left to the readers of this chapter to form their own conclusion concerning the merits of the devices evaluated. Apart from better pressure relief characteristics and skin tissue perfusion, there are many other parameters, such as comfort, cost, ease of use, maintenance and long-term reliability which should be considered before making choice of a support surface for a patient.

Key points

⌘ Technical aspects of support surface performance can be evaluated in the laboratory with differences between support surfaces identified.

⌘ There is no current understanding whether differences in the parameters measured in the laboratory translate into differences in the clinical outcomes achieved using different support surfaces. We simply do not know whether the pressures applied by two surfaces will translate into more pressure ulcers on the surface that applies higher pressure.

⌘ Laboratory-based evaluation should ideally focus upon a range of parameters rather than concentrating upon one (for example, interface pressure) alone.

⌘ Laboratory-based measurements should not, in isolation, influence decisions to purchase or deploy specific support surfaces.

References

Anon (1996) Cover story: technologically advanced alternating pressure mattress. *Hospital Equipment & Supplies* **42**: 3

Bedford PD, Cosin LZ, McCarthy TF, Scott, BO (1961) The alternating pressure mattress. *Gerontologica Clinica* **3**: 69–82

Berjian RA, Douglas HO, Holyoke ED, Goodwin RN, Priore RL (1983) Skin pressure measurements on various mattress surfaces in cancer patients. *Am J Phys Med* **62**: 217–26

Bliss MR, Thomas JM (1992) Randomised controlled trials of pressure reliving supports. *J Tissue Viability* **2**: 89–95

Bliss MR, Thomas JM (1993) An investigative approach: An overview of randomised controlled trials of alternating pressure supports. *Prof Nurse* **8**: 437–44

Bliss MR, Thomas JM (1993) Clinical trials with budgetary implications: Establishing randomised trials of pressure-relieving aids. *Prof Nurse* **8**: 292–6

Clutton-Brock TH, Rithalia SVS (1984) Transcutaneous carbon dioxide monitoring. *Br J Hosp Med* **31**: 225–9

Colin D, Abraham P, Preault L, Bregeon C, Saumet JL (1996) Comparison of 900 and 300 laterally inclined positions in the prevention of pressure ulcers using transcutaneous oxygen and carbon dioxide pressures. *Adv Wound Care* **9**: 35–8

Dunford C (1991) A clinical evaluation of the Nimbus dynamic flotation system. *J Tissue Viability* **1**: 75–8

Exton-Smith N (1987) The patient's not for turning. *Nurs Times* **83**: 42–4

Fletcher J, Billingham G (1993) Mattress replacements: assessment and evaluation. *J Tissue Viability* **3**: 123–6

Gardner WJ, Anderson RM (1948) Alternating pressure alleviates bedsore. *Modern Hospital* **71**: 72–3

Grant LJ (1981) Interface pressure measurement between a patient and a support surface. *MRCOG4* **1**: 7–9

Green MF (1976) The team approach. *Nurs Times* **7**: 292–4

Guttmann L (1976) The prevention and treatment of pressure sores. In: Kenedi RM, Cowden JM, Scales JT, eds. *Bedsore Biomechanics*. University Park Press, Baltimore: 153–9

Hibbs PJ (1988) The economics of pressure sore prevention. *Decubitus* **1**: 32–8

Hussain T (1953) Experimental study of some pressure effects on tissue, with reference to bed-sore problem. *J Pathol Bacteriology* **66**: 347–58

Lockyer-Stevens N (1994) A developing information base for purchasing decisions: a review of pressure-relieving beds for at-risk patients. *Prof Nurse* **9**: 534–42

Maklebust JA, Mondoux L, Sieggreen M (1986) Pressure relief characteristics of various support surfaces used in prevention and treatment of pressure ulcers. *J Enterostomal Therapy* **13**: 85–9

Mayrovitz HN, Smith J (1998) Heel-skin microvascular blood perfusion responses to sustained pressure loading and unloading. *Microcirculation* **5**: 227–33

Mayrovitz HN, Sims N, Taylor MC, Dribin L (2003) Effects of support surface relief pressures on heel skin blood perfusion. *Adv Skin Wound Care* **16**: 141–5

McLeod AG (1997) Principles of alternating pressure surfaces. *Adv Wound Care* **10**: 30–6

McCollumn PT, Spence VA, Walker WF (1986) Oxygen induced changes in the skin as measured by transcutaneous oxymetry. *Br J Surg* **73**: 330–1

Newson TP, Rolfe P (1982) Skin surface PO_2 and blood flow measurements over the ischial tuberosity. *Arch Phys Med Rehab* **63**: 553–6

Panel for the Prediction and Prevention of Pressure Ulcers in Adults (1992) *Pressure Ulcers in Adults: Prediction and Prevention. Clinical Practice Guideline No. 3.* Rockville, Md., Agency for Health Care Policy and Research, Public Health Service, US Department of Health and Human Services, AHCPR Publication No 92–0047, May

Price P, Bale S, Newcombe R, Harding K (1999) Challenging the pressure sore paradigm. *J Wound Care* **8**: 187–9

Pring SRP, Millman P (1998) Measuring interface pressures in mattresses. *J Wound Care* **7**(4): 173–4

Redfern SJ, Jeneid PA, Gillingham ME, Lunn HF (1973) Local pressures with ten types of patient support systems. *Lancet* **2**: 277–80

Rithalia SVS (1991) Pressure sores: methods used for the assessment of patient support surfaces. *Clinical Rehabilitation* **5**: 323–9

Rithalia SVS (1995) Comparison of performance characteristics of the Nimbus and Airwave mattresses. *Int J Rehab Res* **18**: 182–5

Rithalia SVS, Gonsalkorale M (1998) Assessment of alternating air mattresses using a time-based interface pressure threshold technique. *J Rehab Res Dev* **35**: 225–30

Rithalia SVS, Gonsalkorale M (2000) Quantification of pressure relief using interface pressure and tissue perfusion in alternating pressure air mattresses. *Arch Phys Med Rehab* **81**: 1364–9

Rithalia SVS, Heath GH (2000) A change for the better? Measuring improvements in upgraded alternating-pressure air mattresses. *J Wound Care* **9**: 437–4

Rithalia SVS, Russell L (2003) Evaluation of alternating pressure air mattresses using a time based pressure threshold technique and laser Doppler micro-vascular perfusion measurements on the heel (Abstract). *European Pressure Ulcer Advisory Panel Review* **5**: 15–16

Robertson J (1987) Counting the cost. *Nurs Times* **83**: 56

Russell L, Reynolds TM (2000) Randomised controlled trial of two pressure-relieving systems. *J Wound Care* **9**: 52–5

Salisbury RE (1985) Transcutaneous PO_2 monitoring in bedridden burn patients: a physiological analysis of four methods to prevent pressure sores. In: Lee BY, ed. *Chronic Ulcers of the Skin.* McGraw Hill Book Company, New York: 189–95

Sideranko S, Quinn A, Burns K, Froman RD (1992) Effect of position and mattress overlay on sacral and heel pressures in clinical population. *Research in Nursing & Health* **15**: 245–51

Tingle J (1998) Pressure sores: counting the legal cost of nursing neglect. *Br J Ther Rehab* **5**: 431–2

Trumble HC (1930) The skin tolerance for pressure and pressure sores. *Med J Aust* **2**: 724–6

Willis J (1996) Flotation beds: Latest developments. *Nurs Times* **92**: 46–8

Wyss CR, Harrington RM, Burgess EM, Masten FA (1988) Transcutaneous oxygen tension as a predictor of success after an amputation. *J Bone Joint Surg* 70-A: 203–7

Xakellis GC, Frantz RA, Arteaga M, Meletiou S (1991) A comparison of changes in the transcutaneous oxygen tension and capillary blood flow in the skin with increasing compressive weight. *Am J Phys Med Rehab* **70**: 172–7

Xakellis GC, Frant RA, Arteaga M, Meletiou S (1991) A comparison of changes in the transcutaneous tension and capillary blood flow in the skin with increasing compressive weights. *Am J Phys Med* **7**: 172–7

8

Collecting pressure ulcer prevention and management outcomes

Michael Clark, Maureen Benbow, Martyn Butcher, Krzys Gebhardt, Gail Teasley and Jim Zoller

This chapter presents the argument that a combination of efficacy and effectiveness is required to assess fully the impact of interventions, such as pressure-redistributing beds and mattresses. The methodology adopted within a multinational, multicentre, prospective, non-randomized cohort study, designed to record the occurrence and characteristics of patients vulnerable to, or with, established pressure ulcers, is described. General demographic data and the characteristics of pressure ulcers experienced by the 2507 UK subjects recruited to the study across four UK hospitals between July 1996 and May 1998 are presented, with pressure ulcers affecting 218 subjects, of whom 100 presented with ulcers on admission to hospital. Fourteen subjects developed severe ulcers, while a further twenty-four were admitted with full-thickness pressure ulcers.

While the level of health service funding continues to receive national political, media and public interest, what these funds buy and the benefits gained by society largely pass unnoticed. At a macro level are health outcomes such as mortality rates and life expectancy, proportionately lower within countries that devote larger proportions of their national income to health?

At the micro level, the most efficient ways for the health service to tackle the prevention and treatment of common complications of illnesses, like pressure ulcers, need to be examined. In recent years, questions relating to the micro level are assumed to be answerable through the conduct, or interpretation, of specific research designs and, in particular, the randomized controlled trial (RCT) (Cullum *et al*, 2004; Clark, 1996, 1998).

RCTs, particularly when synthesized within systematic literature reviews, are often viewed to be the most appropriate way of removing uncertainty over which interventions to fund or adopt into practice. Such confidence in the RCT stems from the design's high internal validity: 'The confidence that the trial design, conduct, analysis and presentation has minimized or avoided biases in its intervention comparisons' (Moher *et al*, 1996).

While a well-designed and well-executed RCT will certainly offer insights into the efficacy of a drug or device, the effectiveness of either type of intervention may not be shown by RCT studies. This may appear contradictory if 'efficacy' and 'effectiveness' are considered to be equivalent terms. However, efficacy relates to the performance of an intervention under ideal conditions, while its effectiveness describes its performance within the real world. RCTs may fail to capture the effectiveness of an intervention through the study's inclusion and exclusion criteria; these may exclude the most problematic wounds and patients with key co-morbidities.

Effectiveness studies reflect the experience of cohorts of patients who have not been rigorously selected against a set of criteria. Such cohort studies aim to capture both the patterns of resource use and the outcomes of the care received by each member of the cohort. While not able to define the efficacy of any intervention, cohort studies may allow description of the likely effectiveness of an intervention when used in the care of patients. These experiments can also provide data required to capture the financial costs of the care received and allow presentation of cost-effectiveness data and even modelling of the use of an intervention within other care settings and patient populations.

It would appear prudent for any evaluation of a health technology, such as pressure-redistributing (PR) beds and mattresses, to be founded on a mixture of efficacy and effectiveness investigations. When considering the use of PR beds and mattresses, there have been relatively few efficacy studies and fewer of device effectiveness (Cullum *et al*, 2004; Clark, 1998). Perhaps this lack of rigorous effectiveness data relates to the costs of the studies?

Both efficacy and effectiveness studies depend on the reliable and accurate collection of appropriate data, and are likely to incur high data collection costs through the employment of dedicated data collectors. The investment when planning effectiveness studies may be considerable, for large samples may be required 'to allow meaningful statistical interrogation' and, in consequence this 'involves a long-term commitment [which] can be difficult and is frequently costly' (Anon, 1993). With funding from a wound management company a multinational and multicentre study was designed to address issues related to the effectiveness of pressure ulcer prevention and treatment within acute care providers both in the UK and the USA. This chapter describes the methodology adopted in the study along with the number and characteristics of the pressure ulcers experienced by the cohort recruited in the UK. One aim of this chapter is to emphasize that the data collected was broadly comparable to that obtained in previous pressure ulcer epidemiology studies conducted in the UK acute care setting (Clark and Cullum, 1992; Clark and Watts, 1994).

Methodology

This multinational, multicentre, prospective, non-randomized cohort study followed the fate of newly admitted inpatients to wards across five acute care hospitals, four located in the UK and the final site in the USA.

In the UK, the hospitals represented a convenience sample and covered a teaching hospital in London and non-teaching sites in the south-east, south-west and the Midlands. In the USA, data were collected within an acute care provider located in the New York metropolitan area (this data is not reported in this chapter with the focus being upon UK data only). In the UK, eligible subjects were over sixteen years old, able to provide informed consent (or where assent of relatives or appropriate medical staff was available), remained in hospital for at least two days and were not admitted to the following medical specialties: psychiatry, ophthalmology, gynaecology, paediatrics, obstetrics and mental illness. This study was submitted to and approved by the relevant research ethics committees.

Subjects were recruited in the UK by ten data collectors. Nine of these were registered nurses, with the final data collector drawn from a clinical audit department. Three data collectors were assigned to each of the hospitals, with a single data collector available within the south-east site (where data was collected for six months only). All data collectors met at three-month intervals to resolve issues of pressure ulcer classification, risk assessment and provide a formal estimate of their reliability when measuring pressure ulcer dimensions. This last point was assessed through measurement of a set of three-dimensional wound models. Within each NHS trust that participated in this study, site facilitators (the local tissue viability nurse specialist) assisted the access of data collectors to clinical areas. Data collection was organized in a different manner in the USA, where the primary source of data was derived from prospective reviews of medical and nursing records.

Before the commencement of data collection, it was expected that each data collector had to recruit 300 subjects in twelve months. Recruitment was then stratified to reflect the number of patients admitted to each medical specialty, along with the vulnerability of these patients to developing pressure ulcers (Waterlow, 1985). In this study, a Waterlow score below 10 was considered 'minimal risk', 10–14 'low risk', 15–19 'high risk' and scores of 20 or above denoted 'very high risk'. Stratification was based upon the number of admissions and risk scores collected over the six-month period that preceded data collection. Upon calculation of the required number of, for example, high-risk orthopaedic patients, a convenience sample of subjects was recruited up to the predetermined total.

All data were entered directly on to a relational database (Microsoft FoxPro 2.6). Each data collector was not only provided with a laptop computer, but also maintained written records in the event of a catastrophic failure of the laptop and/or program files.

On admission to the study, a unique identification code was generated for each subject. This code allowed the retrieval of previous assessments entered for each subject within the database. Subjects' names were not entered into the database. On admission to the study, the age and sex of each subject, their height and weight, along with the medical problems that prompted the admission to hospital and any associated co-morbidities (coded using ICD-9, the 9th version of the International Classification of Disease, World Health Organization). Data were also collected on admission about the subjects' continence status, appetite, medications, history of previous pressure ulcers, current vulnerability to ulcers and present or previous history of smoking.

Within the UK only, skin condition was assessed using the Arnold skin assessment tool that provides a subjective rating of skin colouration, local circulation, moisture, tone and ability to respond to stimuli (Arnold, 1994). Additionally, the UK data collectors also collected the following items that were not available to the USA investigators: mobility while in bed and when seated was assessed using the Nursing Practice Research Unit mobility assessment tool (Clark and Farrar, 1991; Clark *et al*, 1991). Each subject's physical dependency was assessed using the Barthel score (Mahoney and Barthel, 1965), while an overall quality of life rating was recorded using the thirty-six-item short-form health survey (SF-36) instrument (Ware *et al*, 1993). The comfort of each subject in bed was assessed using the general comfort rating (Shackel *et al*, 1969).

Where subjects were recruited with established ulcers, the number, anatomical location and severity of each ulcer was recorded. In this study, the severity of pressure ulcers was described where a grade I ulcer marks an area of non-blanchable erythema (Clark and Cullum, 1992). Where the skin was broken, each ulcer was observed and classed as either:

- Grade II: superficial break in the skin
- Grade III: destruction of the skin (without cavity)
- Grade IV: destruction of the skin (with cavity).

Within this chapter, grade I and II ulcers are described as superficial ulcers, whereas grade III and IV ulcers are considered to be severe. The maximum length and width of each ulcer was measured from tracings of the wound surface made on to transparent film (McCulloch, 1995; Plassman, 1995). This method provided the greatest precision among other forms of area measurement available in routine clinical practice (Plassman, 1995). The depth of each severe pressure ulcer was measured through the insertion of a sterile cotton-tipped applicator into the ulcer until the applicator made contact with the wound bed (McCulloch, 1995).

The nursing care that subjects received relating to pressure ulcer prevention and management was also documented. The information recorded is listed in *Table 8.1*. Each subject was assessed daily and any changes in the following data recorded: vulnerability to the development of pressure ulcers; the condition of the skin; the condition of any pressure ulcers; and the care received by the subject.

Table 8.1: Documented nursing care that subjects received in relation to pressure ulcer prevention and management
The frequency of physical repositioning in bed, while seated, and the total time each subject spent out of bed each day
The use of urninary catheters and other continence devices
The application of wound dressings or topical applications to intact skin
The use of sheepskin and foam heel and elbow pads
The allocation of patient support surfaces to redistribute pressure while in bed and when seated
The condition of patient support surfaces (denoted by visible malfunctions of electrically powered devices or any deterioration in foam-based devices)
The method and frequency of wound debridement
The use of wound cleansers and wound dressings on established ulcers
The duration of any period passed in accident and emergency
The duration of any surgical procedures (including time in preoperative and postoperative recovery) and the support surfaces used in each setting

All subjects remained in the study until they left hospital, died, or withdrew for any other reason. All data were analysed using the statistical package for the social sciences, software package SPSS Version 8.0 (SPSS Inc, USA).

Demographic and pressure ulcer data

In the UK, 2507 subjects were recruited between 12 July 1996 and 31 May 1998. These subjects were drawn from four acute care providers (*Table 8.2*) with the Midlands site providing 50% of the population. Subjects ranged in age from sixteen to one hundred and three years (median age sixty-nine years), with 55% (*n*=1380) being female. All except sixty subjects were Caucasian (*n*=2446) (one was of unknown ethnic group). The median duration of hospital stay was eight days (range 3–243 days), with 34% (*n*=854) admitted to general medical wards (*Table 8.3*). On discharge from hospital, most subjects (*n*=2108; 84%) returned to their own homes, with 139 discharged to a nursing home. Fifty-nine subjects (2%) died during their stay in hospital.

Table 8.2: Subject demographic information and pressure ulcers

	Hospital location			
	Midlands	South-east	South-west	London
Number recruited	1254	77	655	521
Age (mean; range)	64.57 (16–97)	71.03 (16–99)	66.74 (16–100)	64.46 (17–103)
Sex (male: female)	547:707	24:53	291:364	265:256
Ulcers developed	53	12	31	22
Ulcers present on admission	58	3	22	17

Twenty-nine per cent of subjects (*n*=727) were considered to be at minimal risk of developing pressure ulcers, as judged by the maximum Waterlow score recorded during their stay in hospital. However, 23% (*n*=576) and 19% (*n*=470) of subjects were considered to be at high or very high risk respectively.

Two hundred and eighteen (9%) subjects either developed ulcers after admission (*n*=118 [54%] present for 3613 patient-days), or entered hospital with established pressure ulcers (*n*=100, present for 1917 patient-days). Subjects without ulcers stayed in hospital for 24081 patient-days. The incidence of new ulcers among the study population was 42.6 subjects developing ulcers per 10000 patient-days. Multiple ulcers affected 57 (26%) subjects, with no subject having more than four ulcers. The most severe ulcer experienced by 83% (*n*=180) of subjects either presented as non-reactive erythema (*n*=89) or as a superficial break in the epidermis (*n*=91). Thirty-eight subjects (17%) experienced severe, full-thickness pressure ulcers.

Table 8.3: Medical specialty on admission to hospital

Specialty	Number of subjects admitted
General medicine	854
General surgery	461
Orthopaedics	287
Urology	175
Coronary care	126
Acute care of the elderly	87
Elderly rehabilitation	58
Gynaecology	43
Other	44
Unreported	372

Twenty-four (63%) of the subjects with severe ulcers presented with these wounds on admission to hospital, with four admitted to hospital as a direct consequence of their ulcers (inpatients for sixty-six days).

Overall, the incidence of patients developing severe ulcers was 5.05 patients per 10000 patient-days. Sixty-five per cent of the pressure ulcers affected the sacral area (*n*=141) with the heels being the second most common site (*n*=32). Pressure ulcers were also reported at ten other anatomical sites, with only ten pressure ulcers at sites above the waist.

Fourteen medical problems were the most common reasons for admission to

Table 8.4: Reasons for admission to hospital	
Reason	**Number of subjects admitted**
Chest pain	158
Abdominal pain	153
Carcinoma	107
Dypsnoea	93
Fall	77
Joint replacement	72
Angina	64
Fractured femur	56
Cerebrovascular accident	49
Anaemia	42
Hernia	39
Asthma	38
Congestive cardiac failure	36
Prostate disorders	30
Other reasons	1493

hospital (defined as prompting admission in at least thirty subjects) (*Table 8.4*). Of these, chest (*n*=158) and abdominal (*n*=153) pain along with various carcinomas (*n*=107) were the most frequently recorded reasons for admission to hospital. In 1493 subjects, admission occurred for reasons other than the fourteen most common, with four subjects admitted as a direct consequence of their pressure ulcers. Multiple medical problems were prevalent: 1925 (77%) presenting with at least one co-morbidity. Two hundred and eighty subjects (11%) presented with four co-morbidities. Data on subject height and weight were frequently unavailable with body mass index (BMI) calculated for 2186 (87%) of the population recruited: the median BMI was 24.46 (range 7.03–73.46).

Most subjects were reported to have a good appetite (*n*=1147; 46%), defined as eating at least 75% of the content of all meals. Poor or very poor appetites were recorded in 515 (21%) of the population, where a poor appetite indicated that a maximum of 49% of the meal was eaten. Relatively few subjects were reported to be incontinent, with 108 (4%) and 42 (2%) reported to exhibit urinary or faecal incontinence respectively. One-fifth of all subjects smoked at the time of admission to hospital (*n*=503; 20%).

The range of Barthel scores (at admission) was 0–20 (median 19), suggesting that most subjects were functionally independent (Mahoney and Barthel, 1965). In a similar vein, Nursing Practice Research Unit (NPRU) mobility scores ranged 0–21 (median 0) indicating that most subjects were fully mobile (Clark and Farrar, 1991). However, 206 subjects (8%) were classed as completely immobile (NPRU score of 18 or higher) while 289 subjects (12%) were classed as being dependent on some, if not all, of their physical activities (defined here as a Barthel score of 9 or less).

General vulnerability to developing pressure ulcers was assessed using the Waterlow scale (Waterlow, 1985). Using this tool, 29% of the population (*n*=725) were considered to be at minimal risk of developing ulcers (Waterlow score of under 10). There were 727 (29%) subjects at low risk (Waterlow 10–14), 576 (23%) at high risk (Waterlow 15–19) and finally 470 (19%) at very high risk (Waterlow 20 and above).

Considering subjects' level of activity, most were reported to be fully ambulant (*n*=816; 33%) or partially ambulant (*n*=1081; 43%). The remaining subjects were either confined to bed (*n*=332; 13%) or confined to bed and their chair (*n*=262; 10%). The level of activity of the final sixteen subjects was unreported. While in bed, 2153 (86%) were able to control and alter their posture. One hundred and five subjects (4%) received regular repositioning by nursing staff, while 164 (7%) immobile subjects could not be repositioned because of their medical condition.

Among those not confined to bed, only thirty-one (1%) were regularly repositioned while seated with a further seventy-four immobile seated subjects not repositioned because of their underlying medical problems. The majority (*n*=1996; 80%) of subjects were able to control and adjust their posture. Many subjects were referred to physiotherapists (*n*=656; 26%) with mobility-enhancing aids (of a variety of types) allocated to 637 (25%).

Six hundred and eighty-four subjects (27%) entered hospital through the accident and emergency (A&E) department, with the median stay in A&E being two hours (range 0.02–21.00 hours). Surgical procedures were also commonly experienced by the cohort with 572 (23%) undergoing surgery, the median duration of surgery being 1.3 hours (range 0.08–31 hours).

The 2507 subjects recruited in the UK were provided with a variety of interventions intended to assist both pressure ulcer prevention and treatment. The 105 and thirty-one subjects who were regularly repositioned by nursing staff while in bed or when seated respectively were most commonly assisted at two-hourly intervals (*n*=53 in bed and *n*=16 when seated). Of the 1997 subjects where the duration of chair sitting each day was known, the majority (*n*=772; 39%) sat for between four and eight hours each day. Only 21% (*n*=417) of seated subjects sat for under two hours each day.

Despite lengthy periods sitting in chairs, only 27% (*n*=547) subjects were allocated a PR seat cushion (*Table 8.5*). Thirty-five subjects were allocated alternating pressure air cushions with 275 (14%) allocated some form of foam cushion. The use of pillows and sheepskin fleeces to protect seated subjects was relatively rare, with fifty-two and six subjects allocated such aids respectively. Sixty subjects experienced one change of PR cushion during their stay in hospital, with no subject experiencing use of more than two PR cushions during their stay. Where PR cushions were used the median duration of use was nine days (range 1–229 days).

Table 8.5: Allocation of pressure-redistributing cushions on admission to hospital	
Cushion allocated	**Number of subjects provided**
Foam cushion	333
Adjustable seat	72
Pillow	52
Alternating pressure cushion	35
Fibre-filled cushion	28
Air-filled cushion	8
Sheepskin	6
Other	13
None	1628
Confined to bed	332

The use of wound dressings and skin lotions to delay the onset of pressure damage was rare with twenty-four and 166 subjects allocated these interventions respectively. Film dressings were most commonly used to delay pressure damage (*n*=14) with hydrocolloids used in five cases and a PR dressing on one subject. Most subjects who experienced the use of skin lotions received applications of moisturizing creams (*n*=145; 87%). Only eighteen and three subjects respectively were provided with heel or elbow pads to protect these anatomical sites.

Where subjects had established pressure ulcers (*n*=218), the dressings applied to the ulcers were unreported in fifty-one cases (23%) with no dressing applied in a further forty-nine (22%) subjects (thirty-one uncovered ulcers presented as non-blanching erythema). In eighteen subjects no dressing was applied to ulcers involving breaks to the skin, including one full-thickness ulcer. Where dressings were used, hydrocolloid and film dressings were the most commonly encountered categories (*Table 8.6*). In forty-eight

Table 8.6: Allocation of dressings to established pressure ulcers	
Dressing allocated	**Number of subjects provided**
Hydrocolloid	63
Film dressing	34
Alginate	11
Other	5
N-A dressing	4
Charcoal dressing	1
None	49
Unrecorded	51

Table 8.7: Allocation of pressure-redistributing beds and mattresses on admission to hospital	
Mattress allocated	**Number of subjects provided**
Low pressure foam mattress	961
Standard mattress	639
Static overlay	418
Other	145
Alternating pressure mattress replacement (category 6*)	66
Alternating pressure mattress overlay	78
Alternating pressure mattress replacement (category 7*)	47
Low air loss mattress	3
Air-fluidized bed	1
Unreported	149

*Clark and Rowland, 1989

subjects (22%) at least one change of dressing type occurred during their stay in hospital.

Most subjects were provided with a PR mattress upon admission to hospital, with only 25% (*n*=639) nursed upon standard mattresses (*Table 8.7*). The mattress allocated to 294 subjects (12%) at the time of admission was unrecorded. Primarily, subjects were nursed upon low pressure foam mattresses (*n*=961; 38%). The use of alternating pressure air mattresses was relatively common, with seventy-eight subjects allocated an alternating overlay, sixty-six an alternating replacement mattress (category 6; Clark and Rowland, 1989) and forty-seven provided with a category 7 alternating replacement mattress (Clark and Rowland, 1989). Four other powered PR surfaces were used (one air-fluidized bed and three low-air-loss mattresses). Bedding was reported to be tightly tucked around the bed mattress in 868 (35%) of cases, with tight sheets reported in twelve cases of alternating pressure air mattress use (four overlays, four category 6 and four category 7 dynamic mattresses).

Subjects were often nursed on damaged PR mattresses: 382 were nursed on foam mattresses that failed to provide adequate support (bottomed-out), 377 on stained covers with 123 nursed on breached covers. Fifteen subjects were nursed on dynamic mattresses used in spite of visible or audible alarm signals.

The PR mattress allocated to each subject was frequently changed during the stay in hospital. Two hundred and fifty-seven subjects (10%) experienced one change of mattress type, and two subjects experienced four changes to their bed mattress during their stay. Overall, 2274 (91%) were nursed solely on static support surfaces, 169 solely on dynamic surfaces and the remainder (*n*=64) on a combination of static and dynamic mattresses.

Michael Clark, Maureen Benbow, Martyn Butcher, Krzys Gebhardt, Gail Teasley, Jim Zoller

Discussion

This chapter has argued that the observation and recording of appropriate data on large numbers of subjects may provide information upon resource usage and effectiveness that cannot be captured easily within efficacy studies. This should not be interpreted as an 'attack' on the value of RCTs, reflecting only that such studies should be complemented with other designs that can add to our understanding of the benefits offered by interventions, such as pressure-redistributing support surfaces in the real world of healthcare provision.

In the current study, 2507 subjects were followed through their stay in hospital in the UK. With such a sample size, subsequent analysis and interpretation of the effectiveness of individual interventions within specified patient populations becomes achievable, and will be reported in subsequent publications.

In this chapter we have reported the general demography and characteristics of encountered pressure ulcers, with both the number, distribution and severity to that reported in previous studies (Clark and Cullum, 1992; Clark and Watts, 1994). Subjects were typically elderly females and stayed in hospital for about a week, with no subject staying more than eight months. Over 70% of all subjects were considered vulnerable to developing pressure ulcers, with around 40% at increased risk.

Almost 9% of the cohort experienced pressure ulcers during their stay in hospital, most ulcers having developed after admission. However, most of the severe ulcers were present when the subjects were admitted (Clark and Watts, 1994).

Key points

⌘ Both efficacy and effectiveness studies may be required to assess fully the impact of interventions, such as pressure-redistributing support surfaces.

⌘ A total of 2507 UK adult hospital patients have been followed and the development of pressure ulcers recorded.

⌘ The incidence of pressure ulcers was 42.6 subjects developing ulcers per 10000 patient-days, the incidence of severe pressure ulcers being 5.05 subjects developing per 10000 patient-days.

⌘ Only 27% (n=547) of subjects who sat out of bed during the day were allocated a pressure-redistributing cushion.

⌘ Only 25% (n=639) of all subjects were nursed on standard hospital mattresses, with 191 (8%) nursed on alternating pressure mattresses.

⌘ Many subjects (n=257; 10%) experienced at least one change of mattress during their stay in hospital; two subjects were nursed upon five different mattresses during their hospital stay.

References

Anon (1993) The outcomes agenda. *Outcomes Briefing* 1: 1–2

Arnold N (1994) Clinical study: the relationship between patient perceived risk and actual risk for the development of pressure ulcers. *Ostomy Wound Manage* **40**(3): 36–52

Clark M (1996) Can we evaluate the effectiveness of pressure ulcer treatment without randomized controlled trials? In: Leaper DL, Cherry GW, Dealey C, eds. *Proceedings of the 6th European Conference on Advances in Wound Management*. Macmillan Press, Amsterdam: 124–7

Clark M (1998) Removing the 'estimates and guesses' from practice — evidence-based tissue viability. *J Tissue Viabil* **8**(2): 3–5

Clark M, Cullum N (1992) Matching patient need for pressure ulcer prevention with the supply of pressure-redistributing mattresses. *J Adv Nurs* **17**: 310–6

Clark M, Farrar S (1991) Comparison of pressure ulcer risk calculators. In: Harding KG, Leaper DL, Turner TD, eds. *Proceedings of the 1st European Conference on Advances in Wound Management*. Macmillan Press, Cardiff: 158–61

Clark M, Rowland : (1989) Preventing pressure sores: matching patient and mattress using interface pressure measurements. *Decubitis* **2**(1): 34–9

Clark M, Watts S (1994) The incidence of pressure ulcers within a National Health Service trust hospital. *J Adv Nurs* **20**: 33–6

Clark M, Cullum N, Crow RA, Chapman RG, Farrar S, Rowland LB (1991) *Prevention of Pressure Ulcers: Aspects of the Identification of Patient Vulnerability and the Effectiveness of Preventive Interventions*. Final report to the Department of Health, University of Surrey, Guildford

Cullum N, Deeks J, Sheldon TA, Song F, Fletcher AW (1995) Beds, mattresses and cushions for pressure sore prevention and treatment (Cochrane Review). In: *The Cochrane Library*, Issue 1. John Wiley and Sons Ltd, Chichester

McCulloch JM (1995) Evaluation of patients with open wounds. In: McCulloch JM, Kloth LC, Feeder JA, eds. *Wound Healing: Alternatives in Management*. FA Davis, Philadelphia: 111–34

Mahoney FI, Barthel DW (1965) Functional evaluation: the Barthel index. *Md State Med J* **14**: 61–5

Moher D, Jadad AR, Tugwell P (1996) Assessing the quality of randomized controlled trials: current issues and future directions. *Int J Technol Assess Health Care* **12**(2): 195–208

Plassman P (1995) Measuring wounds: a guide to the use of wound measurement techniques. *J Wound Care* **4**(6): 269–72

Shackel B, Chidsey KD, Shipley P (1969) The assessment of chair comfort. *Ergonomics* **12**(2): 269–306

Ware JE, Snow KK, Kosinski M, Gandek B (1993) *SF-36 Health Survey: Manual and Interpretation Guide*. The Health Institute, New England Medical Centre, Boston

Waterlow J (1985) Pressure sores: a risk assessment card. *Nurs Times* **81**(48): 49–55

9

Debating the relative unimportance of pressure-reducing equipment

Miles E Maylor

This chapter examines some assumptions underlying the provision of pressure-reducing equipment, and argues that failure to 'act first and ask questions later' may be a key source of pressure damage. Indeed, it is argued that prevention of pressure damage can be simplified by identifying three groups of patients: those who have pressure ulcers; those who will develop them if action is not taken; and those who will not get them. The linkage of risk assessment scores and guidelines is challenged as erroneous and misleading.

When asked for an explanation of continuing incidence of pressure ulcers, nurses tend to say that it is the result of lack of preventive equipment (Jones, 1996), lack of nursing knowledge (Russell, 1996), or lack of staff (Olshansky, 1994). However, articles query these aspects: Clark and Cullum (1992) on equipment; Maylor and Torrance (1999a) on knowledge; and Miller (1985) on dependency. Another issue to consider is the bewildering variety of pressure-reducing equipment designed to suit every level of risk. Some organizations have policies and flow charts to guide or direct what should be provided to patients (Waterlow, 1991; Dealey, 1995).

This chapter argues that nurses should be confident and simplify their approach to the allocation of equipment. It is contended that enough is known about equipment for nurses to choose correctly in both preventing pressure damage and encouraging healing, but that nurses often act after damage has already occurred (Bale *et al*, 1995). The consequence of this is unnecessary suffering and expense. Staff are urged to amend policies. Alternating pressure air mattresses should be supplied as soon as a patient is admitted to professional care.

When and where does pressure damage start?

The majority of pressure damage starts in the first few days following admission with an acute episode of illness or enforced immobility (Versluysen, 1985, 1986; Hawthorn and Nyquist, 1988; Gebhardt, 1992; Torrance and Maylor, 1999) (*Table 9.1*). It is not possible to define where patients are most at risk of pressure damage relative to specialties such as orthopaedics or medical wards. The simple reason is that methods of collecting and reporting data differ (eg. incidence as opposed to prevalence, classification of pressure damage, and so forth). Even with the same methodology applied over different departments in a given locality, there are too many preventive and nursing variables to attribute higher or lower prevalence or incidence to particular causes.

There seems enough evidence accumulated from diverse publications to conclude that patients who are acutely ill and immobile are probably the most vulnerable to the effects of unrelieved pressure (Cullum *et al*, 1995; Clark, 1998). This situation is repeated in patients who have undergone major surgery (Armstrong, 2001).

Studies show that community settings, as opposed to the hospital setting, generally have lower prevalence of pressure ulcers (Oot-Giromini, 1993; Meehan, 1994; Thoroddsen, 1999). This finding was part of the stimulus to research whether the difference was attributable in part to different expectations of nurses (Maylor, 2001). Among other results, it was found that community nurses have higher value of pressure ulcer prevention and higher knowledge of contributing factors than their hospital counterparts (Maylor, 1999).

Table 9.1: Incidence reports relating time of onset of pressure ulcers (UK samples)

Study	Details	When sores first noted
Versluysen (1985)	283 patients admitted for acute or elective hip operations, 60 of which developed pressure ulcers	17% of patients had a pressure ulcer on admission, 18% had an ulcer preoperatively, 34% developed an ulcer in the first week and a further 24% developed an ulcer in the second week
Versluysen (1986)	Looks at 100 consecutive admissions of patients over 70 years of age, 66 of these patients developed ulcers	11% of the patients had ulcers present on admission, and 48% had developed ulcers by the first and second day in hospital. The maximum number of new cases of pressure ulcers occurred on the day of the operation (20%). Overall, 83% of patients developed ulcers by the fifth day of hospitalization
Gebhardt (1992)	74 patients with a fractured neck of femur were studied over 15 days from admission	None of the patients had pressure ulcers on admission, 12% developed ulcers on the first and second day, 33% developed ulcers between the first day and postoperatively

How much faith in equipment?

A good device is only as good as the staff using it. Nurses may put too much faith in equipment, almost believing it to be a substitute for a member of the team (Olshansky, 1994).

Evidence of this was encountered by the author while nursing a patient with paraplegia. The patient had developed osteomyelitis associated with pressure ulcers, and it became obvious that surgery was required. The patient was persuaded to go into hospital. However, despite being nursed on a low air loss bed the patient developed further pressure damage. The problem lay in putting too much trust in this sophisticated apparatus, despite the patient telling staff it was too hard. The patient died shortly after being discharged home in a worse state than before.

According to strict research evaluation criteria, there is only one study showing that a low air loss bed reduces incidence of pressure ulcers (in an intensive care setting) (Cullum *et al*, 2004).

Proactive or reactive?

It would be erroneous to say that nurses do not know what to recommend for patients at various levels of risk.

Research into control expectancies and knowledge of prevention of pressure damage has shown that, if anything, nurses tend to be over cautious, opting for equipment generally reserved for patients in a higher risk category than needed (Maylor, 1999). Furthermore, several years of prevalence studies highlight that all patients with existing pressure damage are nursed on an appropriate pressure-reducing item (Torrance and Maylor, 1999; Maylor, 2001).

The view that nurses are reactive rather than proactive is supported by Maylor's (1999) triangulation of psychometric tests, knowledge surveys, prevalence and equipment studies (Maylor and Torrance, 1999a,b; Torrance and Maylor, 1999), and also by others (Bale *et al*, 1995; Westrate and Bruining, 1996; Gunningberg *et al*, 2000).

On one occasion the author came across a patient with peripheral vascular disease being nursed on the base-board side of a non-reversible pressure-reducing mattress. The patient admitted it was very hard. Opposite him was a patient, with an inherited muscular disorder, lying on a standard NHS contract mattress with a marbled cover, who had been admitted with an acute illness and was awaiting transfer to another ward. Such mattresses have been condemned for at-risk patients by recent Royal College of Nursing guidelines (Rycroft-Malone, 2000).

The staff dealing with these two patients, both of whom were at similar high risk of pressure damage, claimed that their priority was to deal with the immediate reason for admission, and that the patients would be assessed for pressure ulcer risk when they arrived at the appropriate ward. The value of pressure ulcer prevention, relative to other concerns has been found to be low for the majority of staff (Maylor, 2000).

During a study of Lowthian's (1989) Pressure Sore Prevention Score (PSPS), factor analysis sub-scale scores in a group of patients with chronic illness showed that the length of time patients spent sitting up could explain more of the variance for those who had ulcers than those who did not (Maylor, unpublished data). In a parallel unpublished pressure ulcer incidence study, factor analysis similarly implied that length of time sitting can be a crucial determinant or predictor of pressure ulcer development, further validating the inclusion of that category in PSPS.

On the other hand, for the chronic patients with ulcers (in contrast to those without), less of the variance was accounted for by the amount of lifting up they could achieve. This again infers that encouraging a person to lift up was introduced as part of the treatment strategy. Furthermore, in the pressure incidence study as opposed to the prevalence one of chronic patients, a small increase in the variance was noted (from 20.6% to 23.7%) for poor general condition when a patient developed a pressure ulcer. There was a larger increase in the variance for sitting up (from 32.3% to 42.2%).

Does this indicate that despite a worsening of their condition patients are still tending to sit out of bed for long periods, thus developing pressure ulcers as a consequence (Collins, 2001)?

Recognizing three groups of patients

Nurses' target for patients with pressure ulcers is healing and rehabilitation (Westrate and Bruining, 1996). For these patients there is a need for the best available equipment, at least until they can get themselves out of a bed or chair without assistance. Alternating pressure air mattress replacement systems (APAMs) will, at least, reduce the probability of further damage when used in conjunction with planned and systematic attempts to increase the frequency of gross postural changes (Gebhardt *et al*, 1996).

Although robust randomized controlled trial data are limited, the few studies available support the claim that air fluidized and low air loss beds improve healing rates (Cullum *et al*, 2004). Clinical experience confirms the use of sophisticated APAMs for speeding the healing of existing pressure ulcers (Bliss and Thomas, 1992; Cullum *et al*, 2004). Prolonged sitting on inadequate support surfaces, especially chairs, must be avoided whenever possible (Gebhardt and Bliss, 1994; Collins, 2001).

It is not uncommon to see patients sitting out for many hours next to expensive APAMs, in order to carry out an 'activity' associated with normal life, ie. sitting. This activity could be dangerous in weak patients with existing pressure damage, as it would increase the chances of developing pressure damage.

Patients without pressure ulcers fall into two groups: those who will go on to get pressure ulcers; and those who will not. As mentioned previously, even patients 'protected' by highly sophisticated equipment develop pressure ulcers. There is little or no evidence linking risk levels with types of equipment.

The Royal College of Nursing clinical practice guidelines on pressure ulcer risk assessment and prevention conclude that there is insufficient evidence to support decisions about selection of devices (Rycroft-Malone, 2000). Furthermore, the reliability of pressure ulcer risk assessment scales has been subject to debate (Watkinson, 1996; Maylor and Roberts, 1999). Therefore, local policies and guidelines explicitly linking risk threshold scores with particular types of equipment may be little more than an attempt to impose some means of control over the distribution of limited quantities of apparatus. Such thinking is probably based on rationing of equipment, rather than clinical reality.

Patients who develop pressure ulcers are mostly victims of both their own inactivity and that of local staff. If a nurse was told that a patient is starting to have an attack of ischaemia likely to lead to a deep vein thrombosis, he/she would probably be very quick to intervene. However, this is happening in relation to patients' pressure areas and ulceration is occurring.

Acutely ill immobile patients get pressure damage. When patients are admitted to hospital they are in a vulnerable state. Unfortunately, willingness to argue for the investment in pressure-relieving apparatus on the basis that a patient might develop pressure damage is a difficult position to be put in, particularly if one is not an argumentative type. An explanation to account for the fact that some people are relunctant to face an argument is found in locus of control theory, where 'internals' assume they personally control outcomes, and 'externals' are less proactive (Goodstadt and Kipnis, 1970; Neaves, 1989; Maylor, 1999). One explanation might be that those who tend to be controlling types affect the priorities of their junior staff, while those who believe more in luck actually intervene to save staff from what they imagine to be inevitable (Maylor, 2001).

The personal expectations of care staff and health providers is largely unaccounted for, but has been shown to have important associations with departmental prevalence of ulcers (Maylor and Torrance, 1999b; Maylor, 2000). Paradoxically, the more nurses believe they control pressure ulcer prevention, the higher the departmental prevalence. In addition, the more they think pressure ulcer prevention cannot be controlled, the lower the prevalence (Maylor, 1999).

The 'controllers' in an organization are predominantly 'internals', and they have an influence on many factors that could affect pressure ulcer outcomes, eg. authority over equipment acquisition and setting work priorities. However, the majority of people tend to be 'externals' and are less likely to challenge decisions (Goodstadt and Hjelle, 1973; Ruble, 1976). The relationship between a nurse's personality and preventing pressure damage is only just being elucidated. There is a well founded suspicion that patients develop pressure ulcers because of individual staff traits and group dynamics over the management of pressure ulcer prevention (Miller, 1985; Maylor, 1999).

There is a large group of patients who will not get pressure ulcers. For this group there is consensus that most static pressure-reducing mattresses, other than the NHS standard, are suitable (Rycroft-Malone, 2000), even in the so-called moderate- to high-risk patients (Cullum *et al*, 2004).

Given that most nurses know how to recognize whether a patient is at risk or not (Bostrom and Kenneth, 1992; Hergenroeder *et al*, 1992; Halfens and Eggink, 1995; Wilkes *et al*, 1996; Maylor and Torrance, 1999a), why is there widespread failure to provide suitable pressure relief for the majority of patients? One explanation for this could be that nurses have not succeeded in convincing managers of the absolutely fundamental need to provide good mattresses and seats.

There are anecdotal reports that, in one case, the Commission for Health Improvement insisted that money was spent on such provision. It also sent a letter to an NHS chief executive, pointing out that the National Institute for Clinical Excellence had endorsed the recommendation that no 'at-risk' patient should be put on a standard NHS specification mattress. This had the effect of liberating sufficient funds in a matter of hours (Maylor, 2001).

Conclusion

This chapter has argued that the identification of patients at risk of pressure damage has become too complicated. Confusion reigns because of the misguided idea that risk level and equipment can be linked, often explicitly, through local or nationally recognized policies and guidelines (Waterlow, 1991; Keal, 1994; Dealey, 1995). The contention is that the way of reducing incidence of pressure ulcers is to simplify both patient groupings and equipment provision.

There are three groups of patients: a small number with existing pressure ulcers; another small number of patients who will go on to develop ulcers; and a large number of patients who will not get ulcers. The first and second group are likely to be admitted with an acute illness and will not be able to move themselves off a bed or chair, or will have an episode mimicking these two factors (eg. surgery). For them, the strategy should be to use APAMs, starting from the moment of admission to hospital (or intraoperatively and immediately postoperatively if they were mobile before surgery).

This should be carried out in conjunction with systematic planned periods of mobilization. For the third group, all that is required is a good pressure-reducing mattress with a two-way stretch cover, as well as mobilization. By doing so, a lot of stress could be taken away from staff trying to apply erroneous and sophisticated pressure damage-reducing guidelines.

Key points

⌘ Patients without pressure ulcers admitted to hospital with an acute illness should be nursed from the outset on a good quality alternating-pressure air mattress.

⌘ When patients can get off a bed or chair unaided, a static pressure-reducing mattress and cushion is likely to be sufficient protection.

⌘ Nursing judgment needs to protect patients proactively, rather than just react when damage has started.

⌘ Linking equipment provision to risk assessment scores is misleading.

References

Armstrong D (2001) An integrative review of pressure relief in surgical patients. *AORN J* **73**(3): 645–8

Bale S, Finlay I, Harding K (1995) Pressure ulcer prevention in a hospice. *J Wound Care* **4**(10): 465–8

Bliss M, Thomas J (1992) Randomized controlled trials of pressure-relieving supports. *J Tissue Viabil* **2**(3): 89–95

Bostrom J, Kenneth H (1992) Staff nurse knowledge and perceptions about prevention of pressure ulcers. *Dermatol Nurs* **4**(5): 365–8

Clark M (1998) Repositioning to prevent pressure ulcers — what is the evidence? *Nurs Stand* **13**(3): 58–64

Clark M, Cullum N (1992) Matching patient need for pressure ulcer prevention with the supply of pressure redistributing mattresses. *J Adv Nurs* **17**(3): 310–16

Collins F (2001) Sitting: pressure ulcer development. *Nurs Stand* **15**(22): 54–8

Cullum N, Deeks J, Fletcher A *et al* (1995) The prevention and treatment of pressure ulcers: how effective are pressure-relieving interventions and risk assessment for the prevention and treatment of pressure ulcers? In: *Effective Health Care Bulletin*. NHS Centre for Reviews and Dissemination, University of York

Cullum N, Deeks J, Sheldon T, Song F, Fletcher A (2004) Beds, mattresses and cushions for pressure sore prevention and treatment. Cochrane Review. The Cochrane Library, Issue 1. John Wiley and Sons Ltd, Chichester

Dealey C (1995) Mattresses and beds: a guide to systems available for relieving and reducing pressure. *J Wound Care* **4**(9): 409–12

Gebhardt K (1992) Preventing pressure ulcers in orthopaedics. *Nurs Stand* **6**(23): S4–S6

Gebhardt K, Bliss M (1994) Preventing pressure ulcers in orthopaedic patients — is prolonged chair nursing detrimental? *J Tissue Viabil* **4**(2): 51–4

Gebhardt K, Bliss M, Winwright P, Thomas J (1996) Pressure-relieving supports in an ICU. *J Wound Care* **5**(3): 116–21

Goodstadt B, Kipnis D (1970) Situational influences on the use of power. *J Appl Psychol* **54**: 201–7

Goodstadt B, Hjelle L (1973) Power to the powerless: locus of control and the use of power. *J Pers Soc Psychol* **27**(2): 190–6

Gunningberg L, Lindholm C, Carlsson M, Sjoden PO (2000) The development of pressure ulcers in patients with hip fractures: inadequate nursing documentation is still a problem. *J Adv Nurs* **31**(5): 1155–64

Halfens R, Eggink M (1995) Knowledge, beliefs and use of nursing methods in preventing pressure ulcers in Dutch hospitals. *Int J Nurs Stud* **32**(1): 16–26

Hawthorn P, Nyquist R (1988) The incidence of pressure ulcers amongst a group of elderly patients with fractured neck of femur. *Care Sci Practice* **6**(1): 3–7

Hergenroeder P, Mosher C, Sebo D (1992) Pressure ulcer assessment — simple or complex? *Decubitus* **5**(14): 42–7

Jones B (1996) Reducing the pressure. *Nurs Times* **92**(29): 59–64

Keal J (1994) A means of tying provision with need. Audit of pressure-relieving aids in community-based hospitals. *Prof Nurse* **10**(3): 161–4

Lowthian P (1989) Identifying and protecting patients who may get pressure ulcers. *Nurs Stand* **4**(4): 26–9

Maylor M (1999) *Controlling the pressure: an investigation of knowledge, locus of control, and value of pressure ulcer prevention in relation to prevalence*. University of Glamorgan

Maylor M (2000) Investigating the value of pressure ulcer prevention. *Br J Nurs* **9**(12): S50–S1

Maylor M (2001) Senior nurses' control expectations and the development of pressure ulcers. *Nurs Stand* **15**(45): 33–7

Maylor M, Roberts A (1999) A comparison of three risk assessment scales. *Prof Nurse* **14**(9) 629–32

Maylor M, Torrance C (1999a) Pressure ulcer survey part 2: nurses' knowledge. *J Wound Care* **8**(2): 49–52

Maylor M, Torrance C (1999b) Pressure ulcer survey part 3: locus of control. *J Wound Care* **8**(3): 101–5

Meehan M (1994) National pressure ulcer prevalence survey. *Adv Wound Care* **7**(3): 27–38

Miller A (1985) Nurse/patient dependency — is it iatrogenic? *J Adv Nurs* **10**(1): 63–9

Neaves J (1989) The relationship of locus of control to decision making in nursing students. *J Nurs Educ* **28**(1): 12–17

Olshansky K (1994) Pressure ulcers: no more excuses — assess institutions instead of patients. *Adv Wound Care* **7**(6): 8–12

Oot-Giromini B (1993) Pressure ulcer prevalence, incidence and associated risk factors in the community. *Decubitus* **6**(5): 24–32

Ruble T (1976): Effect of one's locus of control and the opportunity to participate in planning. *Organ Behav Hum Perform* **16**: 63–73

Russell L (1996) Knowledge and practice in pressure area care. *Prof Nurse* **11**(5): 301–6

Rycroft-Malone J (2000) *Clinical Practice Guidelines. Pressure Ulcer Risk Assessment and Prevention*. Royal College of Nursing, London

Thoroddsen A (1999) Pressure ulcer prevalence: a national survey. *J Clin Nurs* **8**(2): 170–9

Torrance C, Maylor M (1999) Pressure ulcer survey: part one. *J Wound Care* **8**(1): 27–30

Versluysen M (1985) Pressure ulcers in elderly patients. The epidemiology related to hip operations. *J Bone Joint Surg* **67**-B: 10–13

Versluysen M (1986) How elderly patients develop pressure ulcers in hospital. *Br Med J* **292**: 1311–13

Waterlow J (1991) A policy that protects. The Waterlow Pressure Sore Prevention/Treatment Policy. *Prof Nurse* **6**(5): 258–64

Watkinson C (1996) Inter-rater reliability of risk-assessment scales. *Prof Nurse* **11**(11): 751–6

Westrate J, Bruining H (1996) Pressure ulcers in an intensive care unit and related variables: a descriptive study. *Intensive Crit Care Nurs* **12**: 280–4

Wilkes L, Bostock E, Lovitt L, Dennis G (1996) Nurses' knowledge of pressure ulcer management in elderly people. *Br J Nurs* **5**(14): 858–65

Section IV
Moving the pressure ulcer debate forward

Pressure ulcers are now beginning to be seen as a significant challenge in healthcare systems, given both their widespread occurrence and economic consequences. This is a significant step forward from the early days where pressure ulcers were often seen as a hidden problem of little or no importance beyond the realms of nursing practice. Although much has been done a great deal of effort and investigation remain to be invested if tomorrow's practitioners are to face a reduced burden imposed by pressure ulceration. We all know what we want to see in pressure ulceration: better understanding of the causes of these wounds; clarity regarding the effectiveness of established and new interventions; and, of course, evidence that pressure ulceration is becoming rarer year by year. This final section tackles two key issues: undertaking pressure ulcer research and the social consequences of pressure ulceration. It is widely accepted that our body of evidence underpinning the selection of effective interventions is limited – how can this be improved? In recent years, much has been written and discussed regarding the need for appropriately sized randomized controlled trials but often there is a tacit acceptance that the design and the execution of such studies do not meet. There is a clear need to reduce this gap between the ideal and the practical but this journey will only be complete when we as healthcare providers and researchers come together to undertake jointly well-designed comparative studies. Such a destination is fully achievable given the will to collaborate and, of course, the resources with which to do so. For many, the destination of multiple well-designed randomized controlled trials lies at the end of the only journey worth undertaking. However, there remains an important role for alternative scientific designs, including the case study. These have been undervalued probably because of their misuse as evidence of intervention effectiveness. While a case study cannot show any intervention is in itself effective, they can highlight new observations and serve as a means of formulating questions for future research. In this section, the case study is discussed as a scientific design in its own right with guidance delivered on the components required to undertake and report sound case reports. Finally, It cannot be ignored that pressure ulcers present significant personal and societal challenges. For this reason, the last two chapters of this book set out issues at a societal level. The first draws upon the data described in *Chapter 8* to build a series of economic models that can elucidate hypotheses for future exploration in clinical studies. Modelling of economic data is relatively rare when considering pressure ulcers but holds the potential for making explicit the choices we face when tackling pressure ulceration. The final chapter discusses pressure ulceration as an example of passive or active neglect. Much has been made of the growing legal involvement in cases of pressure ulceration. It is not the intention of this book to debate the pros and cons of this new trend, however, it is without doubt one of the elements that will shape pressure ulcer prevention and treatment in the coming years.

10

Case study methodology in tissue viability

Carol Dealey

Case studies are often pesented in relation to tissue viability problems. Within hierarchies of evidence, case studies are sometimes seen to be on a par with expert opinion. This chapter examines the case study as a research method and seeks to determine its value in tissue viability research. The term 'case study' denotes a general strategy for research where several methods of data collection are used to provide an in-depth analysis of an individual, group or institution. Three types of case study are used in research: intrinsic, instrumental and collective. All case studies utilize data triangulation within their design, that is, the use of a variety of sources of data within a study. It is one of the major strengths of the case study method. Data sources include documentary data sources, observation and interviews. As in any research, validity and reliability are important in case study methodology; in particular, construct validity, internal validity and external validity. Case studies are potentially vulnerable to observer error and observer bias. Examples are given of potential case studies in tissue viability and their strengths and weaknesses. If undertaken prospectively, with clearly defined multiple sources of data collection and a documented chain of evidence, case studies can add breadth to our knowledge and experience of caring for patients with tissue viability problems.

Introduction

The movement for evidence-based practice promotes the concept that research should underpin decisions made by healthcare providers. Generally, research evidence is graded following a hierarchy of evidence (Scottish Intercollegiate Guidelines Network, 1995). There are several hierarchies which are used and most consider randomized, controlled trials provide the strongest evidence (*Table 10.1*). This poses problems in tissue viability as wound care and wound prevention is a highly complex process and a range of research methodologies is required in order to provide an adequate research base for practice.

Case studies are a recognised method of presenting information about an interesting or unusual case (Springett and Greaves, 1995; Tanner, 1996; Bardwell, 1997; Dzielski, 1999). Case study methodology is not generally considered to be a research method of any particular value and is graded alongside expert opinion in some hierarchies (Dealey, 1999). Part I of this chapter will consider case study design as a research methodology and its value in tissue viability research.

Case study methodology

Robson (1993) provides a useful definition of a case study:

... a strategy for doing research which involves an empirical investigation of a particular contemporary pheno- menon within its real life context using multiple sources of evidence.

Table 10.1: A hierarchy of research evidence
1a Evidence obtained from meta-analysis of randomized controlled trials
1b Evidence obtained from at least one randomized controlled trial
2a Evidence obtained from at least one well-designed controlled trial without randomization
2b Evidence obtained from at least one other type of well-designed quasi-experimental study
3 Evidence obtained from well-designed non-experimental descriptive studies, such as comparative studies, correlation studies and case studies
4 Evidence obtained from expert committee reports or opinions and/or clinical experiences of respected authorities

Clamp *et al* (1994) suggest that the term 'case study' denotes a general strategy for research where several methods of data collection are used to provide an in-depth analysis of an individual, group or institution. Case studies offer the research an opportunity to gain an in-depth knowledge of the individual or group under investigation. Stake suggests (1998) that there are three types of case study used in research. They are intrinsic, instrumental and collective. The purpose of the intrinsic study is to obtain a deeper understanding of the case or phenomenon, thus the case is of primary interest. Here the intention is to use the phenomenon to be studied to provide insight into a particular issue. The collective case study is an instrumental study which is expanded to include several cases. It is sometimes referred to as multiple case studies. Woods (1997) suggests this design is suitable when there is a need to examine the phenomenon under different circumstances.

Triangulation

Triangulation is an important concept within case study design. It is defined as a method of establishing the validity of a researcher's assertions drawn from the data that has been collected (Schwandt, 1997). It allows the researcher to check one source of information against another and, as such, it improves the quality of data analysis and the accuracy of the findings (Robson, 1993). Yin (1993) suggests that the multiple sources should be used in a conferging manner to allow triangulation over the 'facts of the case'. All case studies utilize data trainagulation within their design, that is, the use of a variety of sources of data within a study (Denzin, 1989). Yin (1989) considers the use of triangulation, one of the major strengths of the case study method.

Data sources which may be used in case study methodology

Documentary data sources

Yin suggests (1989) that the use of documentary data sources is likely to be relevant for most case studies. The main benefit from this data is that it can be used to corroborate information from other sources. However, Yin warns that caution should be used when analysing this type of information, if it was written for purposes other than those of the case study.

Observation

Scientific observation has been described as the systematic selection, observation and recording of behaviours or events (Polit and Hungler, 1995). Such observations might include verbal and non-verbal communications or a range of activities. The relationship of the researcher with those being observed is important. The researcher's activities may be overt or covert. Covert observation has been used in anthropological studies where the researcher has infiltrated a group of people and acted as a full member of the group. There are ethical problems in this type of observation and it is rarely used in healthcare research. Overt observation means that those observed are aware of the observation. This may have an impact on the way they behave.

Interviews

Interviews are a method of obtaining information from individuals. They can be structured, semi-structured or completely unstructured (Polit and Hungler, 1995). Structured interviews have the questions set out in a schedule and there are predetermined answers for each one. This format is often also used in questionnaires. For semi-structured interviews, the interviewer has a list of topics that will help to focus the interviewee on a specific area of interest, whereas an unstructured interview is more conversational. The interviewee is allowed to guide the conversation and discourse on whatever he or she wishes. Such interviews are generally recorded using a tape recorder.

Reliability and validity

High quality research should be conducted with rigour. Key to the concept of rigour is validity and reliability. Validity is concerned with questioning whether a researcher is actually measuring what was intended to be measured (Frankfort-Nachmias and Nachmias, 1996). Reliability relates to the repeatability of the findings of a study (Yin, 1989).

Validity

There are a number of aspects of validity that are relevant to the use of a case study methodology: construct validity, internal validity and external validity (Yin, 1989).

Construct validity

Construct validity considers whether the data collection instrument(s) used in a study actually relate to the theoretical concepts underpinning the reseach. Polit and Hungler (1995) consider establishing construct validity in a research study is difficult and challenging. It can be problematic in case-study resarch as there may be insufficient operational measures established by the researcher (Yin, 1989).

There are a number of ways in which construct validity can be established. One example is that proposed by Campbell and Fiske (1959) using a multitrait-multimethod matrix. This method uses both convergence and discriminability. Convergence looks for evidence that several different methods of measuring a construct provide similar results. Discriminability refers to the ability to differentiate the construct being measured from other constructs (Polit and Hungler, 1995). Both these concepts should be considered when judging construct validity.

Yin suggests several strategies to increase construct validity (Yin, 1989):

- use multiple sources of data collection in such a way as to encourage convergence
- establish a chain of evidence
- review of the draft study report by key informants (Yin, 1989).

Internal validity

Internal validity is concerned with assessing whether a causal relationship can truly be discerned between a treatment and an outcome or whether there is merely a spurious relationship. Campbell and Stanley produced a widely used list of 'threats' to internal validity (Campbell and Stanley, 1963) that was added to by Cook and Campbell (1979). The list includes history, maturation, experimental mortality, testing, instrumentation and regression. Internal validity is of particular importance in experimental and quasi-experimental studies. It is of less importance in a descriptive study.

External validity

External validity is sometimes referred to as generalizability. It is concerned with the extent to which the findings of a study can be generalised to a larger population (Frankfort-Nachmias and Nachmias, 1996). For a study to be truly generalizable, the characteristics of the subjects must reflect the chracteristics of the population as a whole. Polit and Hungler (1995) suggest that this can only be achieved randomly selecting subjects from the target population. They also warn of the dangers of subjectivity and limited generalizability of case studies. Yin argued (1989) that case studies depend upon analytical generalization rather than statistical generalization.

Reliability

A good test of reliability is that if another investigator repreated an earlier study in exactly the same way the findings would be the same. It is, therefore, important that good documentation is maintained with as many operational steps as possible (Yin, 1989). Robson (1993) describes possible threats to reliability as subject error, subject bias, observer error and observer bias. Case studies are potentially vulnerable to observer error and observer bias. Observer error may occur if the researcher fails to use a meticulous approach to data collection leading to incorrect conclusions. Observer bias may occur if the researcher either consciously or unconsciously attributes meanings to an observed action based on the researcher's own beliefs. It is also possible for an observer to choose which observations are included or excluded based on the observer's values and beliefs about what is important. The use of a multiple case study design is of benefit in reducing errors. The use of multiple sources of evidence reduces errors. The use of multiple sources of evidence reduces the potential for observer bias.

Analysing case studies

Case studies are analysed by taking all the different data sources and using them to provide supporting evidence for each other (triangulation). For example, a patient may say that his wound is leaking all the time. This statement can be verified by checking the information from the nursing records for the frequency of dressing change. If the records show that the dressing was changed once or twice daily, then it is reasonable to suppose that the wound is exuding heavily. All the information about the case can then be brought together as a coherent whole to form the case report. If multiple case studies have been undertaken, Yin (1989) suggests preparing a case report for each one and then identifying pattern matches which will allow cross-case conclusions to be developed (*Figure 10.1*).

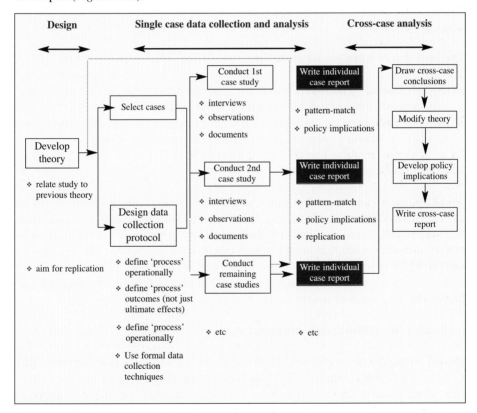

Figure 10.1: Case study method

The use of case study methodology in tissue viability

Intrinsic case studies

Intrinsic case studies are the commonest form of case study used in tissue viability. The case is generally a wound that presents problems to the patient and those providing care. A novel treatment or an interesting response to treatment is usually the motivating force. An example might be a patient with a fungating breast wound. A case study allows the researcher to provide details of the wound and its impact on the patient and her family in some detail and then to progress to the management of these problems. Nelson (2000) has discussed both the strengths and weakness of this type of case study.

The strengths of such case studies are:

- they allow researchers to identify areas worthy of further research
- they allow the development of new hypotheses
- they ensure a greater understanding of the impact of a particular type of wound on the patient.

The weakness of intrinsic case studies are:

- they are frequently retrospective and therefore the information may be incomplete
- they may lack the rigour described earlier in this paper
- they may encourage the adoption of ineffective treatments before they have been subjected to further research such as a randomized controlled trial.

Instrumental case studies

An instrumental case study is undertaken to provide insight into a specific issue. An example of such an issue might be non-compliance of leg ulcer patients. The case would be a patient with a leg ulcer. Such a study is less likely to have some of the weaknesses of the intrinsic case study. It would almost certainly be prospective and have greater validity. There is still the risk of observer error and observer bias. The strength of such a case study is the wealth of detail that can be obtained on a little understood topic that, in turn, can provide direction for further research.

Collective or multiple case studies

The use of multiple case studies enables the researcher to study the same type of case or issue in different circumstances. Using the example of the issue of non-compliance in leg ulcer patients, knowledge can be expanded by studying a housebound patient, a patient who is in full-time employment, a patient who is a full-time carer and so on. Analysis of the results would allow the researcher to identify any patterns leading to cross-case conclusions. Such a study would have greater reliability than a single case study, but only if undertaken with considerable rigour.

Conclusion

Case studies are often seen to have little intrinsic value in tissue viability research. This may be from a lack of understanding of the concepts underpinning case study methodology. If undertaken prospectively, with clearly defined multiple sources of data collection and a documented chain of evidence, they can add breadth to our knowledge and experience of caring for patients with tissue viability problems.

Key points

⌘ Case studies are often used to present new information in pressure ulcer prevention and treatment. At times, case studies are incorrectly used in attempts to position interventions as being effective.

⌘ The case study is a scientific design in its own right and serves to highlight interesting cases and to help formulate questions for future research.

⌘ This chapter sets out guidance for the conduct of case studies demonstrating that when properly conducted and reported the case study does have a role in pressure ulcer research.

References

Bardwell J (1997) Symbiotic relationship of the multidisciplinary team in the management of a patient with diabetic foot ulceration. *J Tissue Viability* **7**: 38–40

Campbell DT, Fiske DW (1959) Convergent and disciminant validation by the multitrait-multimethod matrix. *Psychological Bull* **56**: 81–105

Campbell DT, Stanley JC (1963) *Experimental and Quasi-experimental Designs for Research*. Rand McNally, Chicago

Clamp C, Ballard MP, Gough S (1994) *Resources for Nursing Research*. Library Association Publishing, London

Cook TD, Campbell DT (1979) *Quasi-experimentation: design and analysis issues for field settings*. Rand and McNally, Chicago

Dealey C (1999) *The Care of Wounds*. 2nd edn. Blackwell Science, Oxford: 193

Denzin NK (1989) *The Research Act*. 3rd edn. Prentice Hall, Englewood Cliffs

Dzielski B (1999) From two weeks to twenty-two: one patient's experience of minor surgery. *J Tissue Viability* **9**(1): 17–19

Frankfort-Nachmias C, Nachmias D (1996) *Research Methods in the Social Sciences*. Arnold, London

Nelson EA (2000) The use of case reports in wound care. *J Wound Care* **9**(1): 23–6

Polit DF, Hungler BP (1995) *Nursing Research: principles and methods*. JB Lippincott Company, Philadelphia

Robson C (1993) *Real World Research*. Blackwell Publishers Ltd, Oxford

Schwandt TA (1997) *Qualitative Inquiry: a dictionary of terms*. Sage Publications, Thousand Oaks

Scottish Intercollegiate Guidelines Network (1995) The care of patients with chronic leg ulcer. The Network, Edinburgh

Springett K, Greaves S (1995) Case study: a multidisciplinary team in the management of a patient with diabetic foot ulceration. *J Tissue Viability* **5**: 32–33

Stake RE (1998) Case studies. In: Denzin NK, Lincoln YS eds. *Strategies of Qualitative Enquiry*. Sage Publications, Thousand Oaks

Tanner J (1996) Pustular necrotising angiitis — a personal perspective. *J Tissue Viability* **6**: 15–16

Woods LP (1997) Designing and conducting case study research in nursing. *NT Research* **21**(1): 48–58

Yin RK (1989) *Case Study Research: design and methods*. Sage Publications, Newbury Park

Yin RK (1993) *Applications of Case Study Research*. Sage Publications, Thousand Oaks

11

Models of pressure ulcer care: costs and outcomes

Michael Clark

Pressure ulcer prevention and treatment are expensive with these costs generally believed to be largely avoidable. The consequences for cost-effective treatment are evident. This chapter describes the use of a decision model that predicts both the occurrence and cost of pressure ulcer care within UK hospital populations. The data upon which the model was based was drawn from a large multi-centre cohort study and illustrates the translation of research data into a relevant management tool.

The prevention and treatment of pressure ulcers are not exact sciences; despite effective interventions the final outcome (maintenance of intact skin or complete healing) cannot be predicted with certainty. These uncertainties arise through the interactions between intrinsic biological processes and the complex organisational and care patterns adopted in modern health care.

Organisational (or structural) variables may include the presence of specialist nursing staff and the number of resources such as special beds, while care patterns (process variables) reflect the degree of performance of interventions such as risk assessment and manual repositioning. One strategy for managing the uncertainty inherent in predicting pressure area care outcomes might be to develop models that provide explicit probabilities of achieving certain end-points, such as the complete healing of severe, full-thickness ulcers given the use of particular interventions.

Model building is a relatively recent activity in health care, and perhaps is most commonly encountered when assessing the effect of new pharmaceutical agents (Clark, 1996). Essentially the development of models can be subdivided into a series of three discrete phases; identification of the sub-set of real world events that most strongly affect particular clinical outcomes, determining the probability with which an event influences outcome, and assessing the cost (or consequence) of the outcome.

From this description, model building might be considered as an arcane science with little direct use in daily clinical practice. However, this is not the case for models are used every day in pressure ulcer prevention!

Risk assessment tools

Risk assessment tools are models that attempt to predict clinical outcome. In each tool (or model) a group of risk factors has been identified from among the many possible predisposing intrinsic and extrinsic factors. Each risk factor is then scored to assess its likely contribution to the development of pressure ulcers, with an overall score marking the probability of developing these wounds.

While models are routinely used to infer the likelihood of developing pressure ulcers, these tend to; a) predict outcome at an individual patient level and, b) ignore the likely costs of care. However, these models can be described as decision models given that they predict where intervention may be most beneficial.

Decision models may also allow the economic consequences of care allocation to be predicted; however these economic models are rare in pressure ulcer care. Inman *et al* (1999) described the development of a software-based decision model to evaluate the probable costs of two strategies for allocating pressure-redistributing beds and mattresses.

The data used to allocate probabilities regarding the likely incidence and severity of pressure ulcers that developed while patients were nursed upon the support surfaces was derived from a randomised controlled trial conducted by the authors.

Resource use data (primarily the number of days of use of each support surface) was also gathered through the randomised controlled trial. The costs of the support surfaces were determined based upon whether they would be rented or purchased, with appropriate discount rates and 'useful life' (Conine *et al*, 1990) reported for purchased products.

Inman *et al* (1999) described the use of sensitivity analyses to reflect the robustness of their assumptions regarding mattress cost and longevity, while the perspective of the analysis (that of a hospital administrator) was reported.

The development of the model reported by Inman *et al* (1999) was based upon agreed guidelines for the development and reporting of economic models (Canadian Coordinating Office for Health Technology Assessment [CCOHTA], 1995). The model was used to explore whether costs were lower when purchased or a combination of purchased and rented support surfaces were used in an intensive care unit.

From a concurrent randomised controlled trial the incidence of pressure ulcers was similar within the two groups, and so the model was considered to provide a cost-minimisation analysis. Within realistic limits, the cost of use of the purchased products was lower than the combination of purchased and rented equipment.

This is the sole reported use of decision models to predict the economic consequences of pressure ulcer prevention. Decision models are also rare, at this time, across other aspects of wound care. Parente (1997) modelled the costs incurred through use of skin substitutes or cadaveric tissue in the treatment of burns, while Maxwell *et al* (2000) reported the modelling of deep venous thrombosis prophylaxis in patients experiencing surgery for gynaecologic cancers; in this model external pneumatic compression appeared to be the most cost-effective intervention.

Finally, Schonfeld *et al* (2000) compared the economic impact of treating venous leg ulcers with a skin substitute or compression therapy. In this model, treatment with the skin substitute both reduced the costs of care while increasing the time between successive recurrences of the ulcers.

While economic models have yet to make a major impact upon the evaluation of wound care interventions, certain principles for their development and use are clear. All models extract specific key events or interventions, so they cannot claim to capture all events that may influence outcome, only the most significant.

There is clearly a trade-off between a model's comprehensiveness and its complexity. Models can include multiple events and track patients' movement between states over time (for example, healing followed by recurrence of pressure ulcers); however, as the model approaches 'reality' then its complexity (in mathematical and programming terms) will increase, so obscuring its inherent assumptions and limitations for many users of the model.

As illustrated by Inman *et al* (1999) the probabilities and resource use data used to construct a model should be based upon sound primary data, and not be dependent upon consensus and expert opinion. Sensitivity analysis should be performed to test the robustness of the model's conclusions: are these sensitive to changes in the data used to develop the model? Finally, the perspective of the model should be explicit: does the model mirror costs to society; to the healthcare system; or to an individual care provider, medical speciality or ward (even the individual patient)?

Changing the perspective of the model will have profound consequences for the costs that need to be captured within the model, for example, patients' loss of earnings through developing pressure ulcers may be an important cost to the individual and to society but is largely irrelevant if the perspective is that of a hospital manager.

Development of an economic model predicting the costs of pressure ulcer prevention and treatment

Clark *et al* (*Chapter 8*) have described a multi-national, multi-centre study that followed the fate of cohorts of hospital in-patients with specific reference to the development of pressure ulcers and the healing of established ulcers.

The data gathered from the 2507 UK subjects recruited was used to provide the outcomes (incidence and healing) and resource use (length of use of support surfaces) to develop a decision model comparing the economic effect of different support surface interventions. The model was constructed using decision analysis software (DATA v3.5 for Health Care, TreeAge Software, Inc, Williamstown, MA, USA) with the perspective being that of a hospital manager.

Patients enter the model either with established pressure ulcers or free from these wounds with the relevant proportions derived from the multi-centre study (*Figure 11.1*). Where patients enter with established ulcers, these can be either superficial (grades 1 and 2; Clark and Cullum, 1992) or severe (grades 3 and 4; Clark and Cullum, 1992).

Patients with superficial ulcers can either be allocated various static or dynamic mattresses, with the dynamic group further broken into mattress replacements or mattress overlays and then into those support surfaces (*Figure 11.1*).

Patients with severe pressure ulcers also were distributed between these forms of support surface, but were also available for surgical repair of their pressure ulcer(s).

The end points, regardless of treatment group, were either ulcer healed or ulcer remains open at the time of discharge from hospital. All non-mattress related pressure ulcer treatment costs (for example, wound dressings) were included as a fixed cost per day of treatment based upon the median cost of the dressings encountered during the multi-centre study. All costs are reported in 1998 figures.

All support surfaces were considered to be purchased, with the per day of use cost based upon the assumed 'useful life' (Conine *et al*, 1990) with straight-line depreciation and constant use of the resource (Clark *et al*, 1993).

Static and dynamic mattresses were assumed to have a useful life of either one or five years respectively. The potential for costs to be incurred as a result of litigation following the development of severe pressure ulcers upon static support surfaces was also included where appropriate within the model.

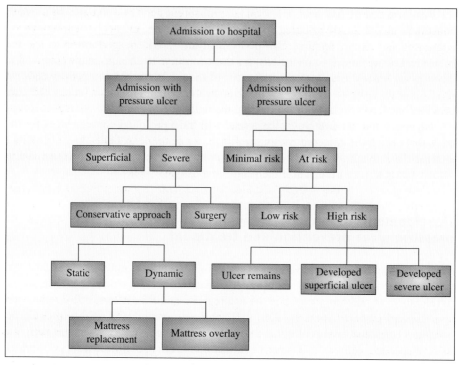

Figure 11.1: Schematic diagram of the structure of the decision model. The use of support surfaces has been omitted from thje prevention arm of the figure with the final end-points shown. The options for support surface use follow the scheme highlighted under severe ulcers present on admission to hospital

The subjects

Where subjects were considered to have entered the model without pressure ulcers, these were distributed between those at minimal risk and those at risk, with risk quantified using the Waterlow scale (Waterlow, 1985).

Where patients were considered at risk of developing pressure ulcers, this group was sub-divided into those at low and high risk. Subjects without pressure ulcers were then allocated dynamic or static mattresses in a similar manner to those who entered the model with established ulcers (*Figure 11.1*).

The end-points for pressure ulcer prevention were either patients remained ulcer free, or developed superficial ulcer or they developed a severe ulcer. All support surface costs along with non-mattress related costs (primarily wound dressings) were subjected to sensitivity analyses in which the median cost per day was varied by +50% and –50%.

Simple modelling

The model is, at this stage, simplistic and does not allow for patients initially ulcer-free, but who develop these wounds entering the treatment arm of the model. This is likely to underestimate the costs of developing pressure ulcers while in hospital for no account is taken of dressing and other costs once a pressure ulcer has developed in a patient initially free of such wounds. Nor have the effects, and costs, of alternative interventions, such as manual repositioning of patients, been considered in the current model.

These simplifications reduce the 'reality' of the model, but do allow the focus to rest upon alternative strategies for mattress allocation. The model was constructed with the assumption that the effectiveness of different interventions was similar; while this may hold true for comparisons between dynamic products, it is unlikely that foam and dynamic mattresses are of equivalent effectiveness.

However, this could not be tested within the available data-set due to the allocation of foam and dynamic products to patients at different susceptibility to developing pressure ulcers, based upon their mobility and Waterlow scores.

Given that the model considers interventions to have similar effectiveness, then all comparisons derived from the model seek to minimise the cost of the intervention used (cost-minimisation analysis).

Optimum treatment

The optimal paths for prevention and treatment, as derived from the model were typically robust to changes in support surface and other costs. Where patients are admitted to hospital with severe pressure ulcers, then conservative treatment was always favoured over surgical repair of the ulcer.

The lowest-cost interventions for the treatment of severe pressure ulcers were considered to be dynamic mattress replacements. This group of interventions was also favoured by the model as the lowest-cost intervention for the prevention of pressure ulcers among high-risk patients.

Where patients were admitted without pressure ulcers and at minimal or low risk of developing such wounds, then foam mattresses provided the lowest-cost intervention. Dynamic mattresses were only preferred over foam mattresses when considering the treatment of superficial pressure ulcers present upon admission if the daily cost of use of the dynamic mattresses did not exceed £0.80.

Cost analysis

The model, with its current assumptions and costs, would suggest that the cost of pressure ulcer prevention and treatment would consume £31 per in-patient admission, with costs highest when treating severe pressure ulcers present upon admission (£89 per patient) and when preventing pressure ulcer development among high risk subjects (£88 per patient).

Three successive Monte Carlo simulations were conducted, each following the fate of 100 consecutive new admissions to hospital (*Table 11.1*). From these simulations, the mean cost per patient ranged from £29 to £36, with the median being £9.

The prevalence of pressure ulcers upon admission ranged from 0% to 4%, with a 3% or 4% incidence predicted during the stay in hospital. Over the three simulations, a total of eleven patients were predicted to develop pressure ulcers; of these, eight (72.7%) were expected to be superficial wounds.

Table 11.1: Monte Carlo simulations tracking the pressure ulcers present among three separate cohorts of 100 patients admitted to hospital

	Cohort 1	Cohort 2	Cohort 3
Cost of pressure ulcer care, £ (mean, median, lower and upper range)	29, 9 (2–99)	35, 9 (2–99)	36, 9 (2–99)
Prevalence of pressure ulcer on admission %	4	0	4
Incidence %	4	3	4
Incidence superficial to severe ulcers	3:1	2:1	3:1
Overall prevalence of pressure ulcers among cohort %	8	3	8

Conclusions

The construction of decision models can help elucidate the lowest cost intervention for particular clinical scenarios, and where robust data upon effectiveness is available then the model can be amended to provide comparisons based upon interventions' cost-effectiveness.

The current model of pressure ulcer prevention and treatment, albeit crude and relatively simplistic, has highlighted that use of dynamic replacement mattresses might incur the lowest costs when treating severe pressure ulcers or when preventing these wounds developing among the most vulnerable groups of patients.

Foam mattresses were the lowest-cost intervention when patients presented with minimal or low risk of developing pressure ulcers. These observations were robust with respect to the sensitivity analyses conducted to explore the impact of changing mattress and wound dressing costs.

The model can also be used to predict the likely financial costs of pressure area care given knowledge of the prevalence of ulcers at admission, the vulnerability of the patient population and the incidence of pressure ulcers during the stay in hospital. The model predicts that for every 1000 in-patient admissions pressure ulcer prevention and treatment would consume £31,000 in marginal costs, excluding any prolongation of hospital stay.

The prevalence of pressure ulcers in hospital as predicted by the model ranged from 3–8%, with incidences of between 3–4%, these estimates are not dissimilar from measured prevalence and incidence rates (for example, Clark and Cullum 1992; Clark and Watts, 1994).

Modelling of healthcare processes and outcomes can provide useful insights; however, models depend upon the quality of the data upon which they are constructed. The model described in this chapter was based upon resource use and outcome data gathered during a large prospective cohort study, with data drawn from 2507 UK hospital patients.

Additionally, models should include appropriate sensitivity analyses to test the robustness of any decisions based upon information from consensus or expert opinion. In the current model, the costs of resources were subject to sensitivity analyses with most optimal care paths robust to changing resource costs.

Modelling should be treated with caution for bias would be relatively easy to introduce, but with increasing awareness of 'sound' methods of model construction (for example, the Canadian Coordinating Office for Health Technology Assessment

[CCOHTA], 1995) then healthcare managers, practitioners and consumers can now have greater confidence in the predictions offered by decision models.

Key points

⌘ Pressure ulcer outcome data can be used to investigate the economic impact of the decisions we make regarding how best to prevent or treat pressure ulcers.

⌘ Economic modelling represents a rapidly growing field in health outcomes research and is subject to criteria that ensure the quality of the model and its predictions.

⌘ Each model needs to trade-off its complexity and its comprehensiveness — a comprehensive model may be simply too mathematically complex for many users.

⌘ The model suggested that the marginal cost of support surface and wound dressing use may be £31000 for every 1000 inpatient admissions. This excludes the cost of nursing time required to reposition manually patients.

References

Canadian Coordinating Office for Health Technology Assessment (CCOHTA) (1995) Guidelines for the economic evaluation of pharmaceuticals: Canada. *Int J Technol Assess Health Care* **11**: 796–7

Clark M, Cullum N (1992) Matching patient need for pressure sore prevention with the supply of pressure-redistributing mattresses. *J Adv Nurs* **17**: 310–16

Clark M, Watts S, Chapman RG, Field K, Carey G (1993) *The financial costs of pressure sores to the National Health Service: A case study. Final Report to the Department of Health.* University of Surrey, Guildford

Clark M, Watts S (1994) The incidence of pressure sores within a National Health Service Trust Hospital during 1991. *J Adv Nurs* **20**: 33–6

Clark M (1996) Can we evaluate the effectiveness of pressure sore treatment without randomized controlled trials? In: Leaper DL, Cherry GW, Dealey C, eds. Proceedings of the 6th European Conference on Advances in Wound Management. Amsterdam. Macmillan Press: 124–7

Conine TA, Daechsel D, Choi AKM, Lau MS (1990) Costs and acceptability of two special overlays for the prevention of pressure sores. *Rehabilitation Nurs* **15**(3):133–7

Inman K, Dymock K, Fysh N, Robbins B, Rutledge F, Sibbald W (1999) Pressure Ulcer Prevention: A Randomized Controlled Trial of 2 Risk-Directed Strategies for Patient Surface Assignment. *Adv Wound Care* **12**: 73–80

Maxwell G, Myers E, Clarke-Pearson D (2000) Cost-effectiveness of deep venous thrombosis in gynecologic oncology surgery. *Obstet Gynecol* **95**(2): 206–14

Parente S (1997) Estimating the economic cost offsets of using Dermagraft-TC as an alternative to cadaver allograft in the treatment of graftable burns. *J Burn Care Rehabil* **18**: 18–24

Schonfeld W, Villa K, Fastenau J, Mazonson P, Falanga V (2000) An economic assessment of Apligraf (Graftskin) for the treatment of hard-to-heal venous leg ulcers. *Wound Repair Regeneration* **8**(4): 251–7

Waterlow J (1985) A risk assessment card. *Nurs Times* **81**: 49–55

12

Pressure ulcers as indicators of neglect

Kieran Walsh and Gerry Bennett

Until recently, pressure ulcers have attracted very little attention from the scientific community. This is changing quickly for a number of reasons, including an increasing awareness of medical responsibility, medical audit and research, cost management and litigation. Pressure ulcers are acute injuries caused by critical ischaemia of the skin. They occur in sick patients with peripheral circulatory failure. Pressure ulcers occur mainly in normal tissue and start to heal as soon as the pressure is relieved. Most pressure ulcers are preventable. They are often the result of medical or nursing negligence when they occur in hospitals or care home settings. Most pressure ulcers can be prevented following careful assessment and the provision of appropriate support surfaces. The majority of ulcers arise because of passive neglect. For example, attention given to risk assessment or to planning appropriate care is often inadequate. Active neglect occurs because of deliberate allowance of harm to the elderly person. Pressure ulcers may be indicative of either form of neglect.

Elder abuse and neglect

Elder abuse and neglect may be defined as a single or repeated act or lack of appropriate action, occurring within any relationship where there is an expectation of trust, which causes harm or distress to an older person (Action on Elder Abuse, 1995). Pressure ulcers may occur as a result of elder abuse or neglect (Nold, 1979). This may occur in hospitals or in nursing homes (Hirschael, 1996). Indeed, the presence of pressure ulcers in care home residents may be the first indicator of abuse or neglect.

Individual care workers may be responsible for the abuse, or the regimen of the care home may be abusive (institutionalized abuse). The acts or omissions which result in abuse may be attributable to a number of factors:

- lack of staff training
- work-related stress
- the organizational culture of the institution
- the character of individual staff members
- the level of dependency of the residents.

It is usually assumed that elder abuse or neglect only occurs in poor quality homes, but in fact, abuse can occur in any home.

Prevalence

Prevalence may be defined as the total number of cases of a disease in a population at one particular time. There is a wide range in the results of prevalence studies of pressure ulcers. A survey in Glasgow showed the prevalence rate to be 8.8% of patients admitted to hospital. A severe pressure ulcer was present in 1.5% of the study population. A study in the Border's health board area found the pressure ulcer prevalence rate in patients acutely admitted to hospital to be 9.4%. Two per cent of these patients had a severe pressure ulcer. Most prevalence studies in the UK indicate that between 8 and 20% of hospital patients have pressure ulcers.

Incidence may be defined as the number of new cases of a disease in a population in a given period. In a study by Bergstrom (1996), the incidence of pressure ulcers was 8% in a hospital setting and 23% in nursing homes. Health care workers should aim to reduce the incidence of pressure sores to 3% or less.

The cost of pressure ulcers to the health service is enormous: pressure ulcers cost an estimated £320 million in 1993 (Audit Commission, 1995). The cost of pressure ulcers is multifactoria: it includes the costs of prolonged hospital stays, use of medications and bandages, additional outpatient appointments, complaints management and litigation. However, there is little knowledge of the prevalence of pressure ulcers in nursing or residential homes in the UK. Reports in the USA indicate that between 20 and 35% of elderly people have pressure ulcers at the time of admission to a nursing home. There are also few research data on the prevalence of neglect in care homes in the UK. Pillemer *et al* (1989) found that 36% of nursing staff in care homes in the USA had observed physical abuse in the home where they worked.

Aetiology

Many factors contribute to the failure of the mechanisms of the body to prevent pressure ulcers. These risk indicators may be divided into intrinsic and extrinsic factors (*Table 12.1*).

Table 12.1: Intrinsic and extrinsic risk factors

Intrinsic	Extrinsic
Acute illness	Long waiting times on hard trolleys
Cardiovascular disease	Hardness of hospital beds
Decreased sensation	Long periods sitting in a chair
Cognitive impairment	Long periods in the operating theatre
Malnutrition	Use of restraints
Paralysis	Inappropriate use of compression hosiery
Peripheral vascular disease	Shearing forces from bedclothes
Failure of vasomotor reflexes	

The following factors may also contribute to the development of pressure ulcers as a result of neglect in care homes:

- use of restraints
- poor nutrition
- poor management of urinary and faecal incontinence
- inadequate mobilization of residents
- inadequate use of pressure-redistributing equipment.

Prevention

All patients admitted to a care home should be assessed for risk factors for pressure ulcers. This assessment should be carried out at the time of admission. It should be repeated if there is any change in the clinical status of the resident. Assessments should be recorded in an individualized care plan. This care plan should be reviewed and regularly updated. Staff should use appropriate assessment scales to predict the risk of developing pressure ulcers. A full examination of pressure areas should be carried out on admission. All patients who are at risk of developing pressure ulcers should be given pressure-relieving support immediately. The at-risk patient should be transferred to an alternating pressure area mattress as soon as possible.

Alternating pressure area mattresses have been shown to prevent pressure ulcers in most elderly patients (Bliss, 1995). The mattresses vary from the inexpensive to the very expensive. Inexpensive mattresses are effective for most patients. In most cases, these mattresses obviate the need for regular turning (except for patient comfort). When moving a patient, staff should lift rather than drag the limbs or body. Wheelchair bound patients should sit on pressure-relieving surfaces. Urinary and faecal incontinence should be treated appropriately.

Patients should eat a healthy diet and should be encouraged to be mobile. Physical restraints should be avoided. Heating pads, blankets and lamps should be avoided as they increase tissue demands for oxygen and nutrients. Good skin care is crucial. The skin should be cleaned thoroughly and moisturizing cream used when it becomes dry and cracked. There is evidence that care homes can succeed in providing at least some of these measures (Kane, 1993).

Pressure ulcers and medical negligence

The essential feature of pressure ulcer management is prevention. Unfortunately, it is in this area that healthcare practitioners fail to perform to adequate standards. Ninety-five per cent of pressure ulcers are preventable with proper early management (Hibbs, 1987). Medical and nursing staff must take responsibility for this aspect of care. Pressure ulcers are likely to be an increasing cause of claims for compensation. They are also likely to become an important parameter in clinical audit and quality (Banks, 1998).

The best way to prevent pressure ulcers is to promote excellence in pressure ulcer prevention. All healthcare workers in all specialities and settings should be able to recognize susceptible patients and provide appropriate treatment. Pressure care nurse specialists should be appointed in every district. Cost-effective and up-to-date pressure-redistributing equipment should be available in all care home settings. Equipment should be available twenty-four hours a day and should be serviced regularly. Care workers should attend in-service training sessions in pressure area care. The decision about whether to use pressure-relieving equipment should form part of the treatment plan of all patients.

In reality, these standards are often not met. The Audit Commission (1995) found serious lapses in the way pressure ulcer prevention is carried out (Health Care Risk Report, 1996). Problems include poor standards in assessment and prevention. Record-keeping and communication with patients and relatives are often substandard. In many cases, there is no evidence of pressure ulcer risk assessment in the case notes.

Pressure-relieving measures are often only instituted once tissue damage has occurred. Nutritional assessments are infrequently undertaken. Grossly negligent medical and nursing practices have been identified in some cases (Tingle, 1997). In some cases, these lapses have led directly to the death of patients. Frequently, great pain and suffering are also caused. Few hospitals and care homes have a comprehensive approach to care and education in this area.

Treatment

Debridement of superficial wounds should occur naturally. This is encouraged by cleaning the wound with saline and keeping it moist. Dressings should encourage moist wound healing. The effectiveness and adverse effects of a wide range of dressings should be taken into account. Clinical nurse specialists in tissue viability provide invaluable advice in this area.

Pain relief is often neglected but is very important: patients often require opioid analgesia for severe pain. Urinary catheterization is often effective as a temporary measure to ensure that the ulcer is kept clean and dry. Offensive odours should be tackled with frequent dressings, charcoal-containing coverings and occasionally metronidazole. Systemic antibiotics may be indicated if there is cellulitis or systemic infection. Many patients require nutritional supplementation. Vitamin C and zinc may be given empirically as they aid wound healing.

In the occasional patient, surgery may be required if a deep ulcer is present or if an ulcer does not respond to conservative management.

The role of the ombudsman

The ombudsman (health service commissioner) investigates complaints about the clinical judgment of doctors and nurses who work in the NHS (Health Service Commissioner, 1996a). The ombudsman is completely independent of the government and the NHS and may call on health professionals to explain their actions. The ombudsman can make recommendations for change but cannot award compensation.

The ombudsman has investigated complaints involving pressure ulcers. A number of problems with care have been identified:

• inadequate nursing care

- delay in taking preventive measures
- poor standard of record keeping
- unsatisfactory communication with relatives
- inadequate provision of special mattresses
- inadequate education of staff (Health Service Commissioner, 1996b).

It is essential that these shortcomings are overcome and that all patients receive prompt and appropriate pressure area care.

Other remedies to abuse and neglect

First, the occurrence of elder abuse and neglect in care homes should be recognized. It is very likely that the majority of pressure ulcers are never reported, and a greater spirit of openness should be encouraged so that this problem is acknowledged.

There are a number of measures that may be taken which would reduce the risk of abuse. Care homes should have visiting hours for relatives and friends that are more flexible and open. Furthermore, a more open management culture should be encouraged as well as constructive criticism of the service provided as it can be very stressful for a care worker or resident to complain about standards of care. To do so often means to risk dismissal or further neglect. Whistle-blowers should be protected from these punitive actions.

Nursing and residential homes should be subject to regular monitoring and should have open and explicit complaints procedures. Complaints should be dealt with speedily and openly, and the results of the investigation into a complaint should be made available to all parties as soon as possible. An apology should be made to patients and relatives when appropriate. Lessons must be learnt from complaints. Staff should be educated about pressure ulcers and elder abuse and neglect. All staff should be adequately supervised.

Inspection and registration units also have an important role to play in protecting elderly residents from neglect. They may visit a home as part of an annual inspection process or to investigate specific complaints. Inspectors may also pick up early indicators of abuse within a care home, such as a poor atmosphere within the home, and thus prevent an abusive situation from worsening. If a complaint is made to a registration unit about a patient who has developed a pressure ulcer, the unit should assess how the incident is being handled. If necessary, it should conduct its own investigation to decide if any breach of registration has occurred.

Research has shown that patients know little about pressure ulcers. Yet when they are asked, patients are eager for more information. Patients and their informal carers should be given written information on the causes and prevention of pressure ulcers (Benbow, 1996).

Conclusion

A survey of medical schools in the UK revealed that medical education in wound care is inadequate for doctors' clinical and medicolegal needs (Bennett, 1992). This situation must be remedied. Knowledge of pressure area care should be examined routinely in undergraduate and postgraduate medical and nursing examinations.

GPs must play a key role in pressure ulcer prevention in the community. Pressure ulcers frequently result from negligent care. The best way to prevent pressure ulcers is to promote excellence in pressure ulcer prevention. Ninety-five per cent of pressure ulcers are preventable with proper, early management.

Key points

⌘ Awareness of the personal and societal cost of pressure ulcers is growing and has resulted in claims for damages where pressure damage has been sustained.

⌘ This chapter introduces pressure ulcers and the failure of prevention within the wider context of the care of elderly people.

⌘ It may be emotive to equate pressure ulcer occurence with passive or active neglect, however, this association well illustrates the growing complexity of the potential repercussions following pressure ulcer development.

References

Action on Elder Abuse (1995) *Everybody's Business: Taking Action on Elder Abuse*. Action on Elder Abuse, London

Audit Commission (1995) *United They Stand: Coordinating Care for Elderly Patients with Hip Fracture*. HMSO, London

Banks V (1998) Management issues in pressure area care. *J Wound Care* **7**(7): 369–70

Benbow M (1996) Pressure sore guidelines: patient/carer involvement and education. *Br J Nurs* **5**(3): 182–7

Bennett GCJ (1992) Teaching of wound care to medical undergraduates (results of a UK national survey). *J Tissue Viability* **2**: 50–1

Bergstrom N, Braden B, Kemp M, Champagne M, Ruby E(1996) Multi-site study of incidence of pressure ulcers and the relationship between risk level, demographic characteristics, diagnoses and prescription of preventive interventions. *J Am Geriatr Soc* **44**(1): 22–30

Bliss MR (1995) Preventing pressure sores in elderly patients: a comparison of seven mattress overlays. *Age Ageing* **24**: 297–302

Health Care Risk Report (1996) Case reviews, care of the elderly. *HCRR* **2**(10): 2–3

Health Service Commissioner (1996a) *A Guide to the work of the Health Service Ombudsman*. HSC, London

Health Service Commissioner (1996b) Fourth Report for Session 1995-6. Annual Report for 1995–96. HMSO, London

Hibbs PJ (1987) Prevention: Can we afford it? The third Pressure Sore Symposium. Bath, 11-12 March, 1987

Hirschael AE (1996) Setting the stage: the advocate's struggle to address gross neglect in Philadelphia nursing homes. *J Elder Abuse and Neglect* **8**(3): 5–20

Kane RL, Williams CC, Williams TF, Kane RA (1993) Restraining restraints: changes in a standard of care. *Annu Rev Public Health* **14**(5): 545–84

Nold O (1979) Consequences of neglect: established bed sores. *Soins* **24**(11): 33–41

Pillemer KA, Moore DW (1989)` Abuse of patients in nursing homes: findings from a survey of staff. *Gerontologist* **29**(3): 314–20

Tingle J (1997) Pressure sores: counting the legal cost of nursing neglect. *Br J Nurs* **6**(13) 757–8

Conclusion

This book began with chapters upon pressure ulcer epidemiology and it is to this vital issue that we must return within these concluding remarks. While UK health care providers are continually pressed for data upon the number of patients affected and the severity of their pressure ulcers, there is no clear guidance upon how such audits are to be conducted, reported and interpreted. The continued failure to provide such a framework for pressure ulcer audits is unacceptable and there is an urgent need for the general acceptance that a systematic approach to audit must be a priority.

A call for formal guidance upon pressure ulcer audit should not be confused with any effort to use pressure ulcers as indicators of the quality of healthcare delivery. It may be that some pressure ulcers mark the delivery of poor quality care, but it is equally obvious that not all pressure ulcers result from deficits in our practice. There are simply too many gaps in our awareness of pressure ulcer aetiology to accept such simplistic statements that pressure ulcer prevalence or incidence is an unambiguous indicator of the quality of care. Let us move forward from using pressure ulcer occurrence as an indicator of quality and rather let us seek to use systematic audit as a measure of our success or failure in tackling this group of wounds.

Many would say: but should we record pressure ulcer prevalence, incidence or incidents? Others might add: but how do we take account of changes in the characteristics of our patient populations? These are technical issues that could be answered if we, as a wound care community, had a common will to resolve these epidemiological challenges. That systematic audit can be achieved is not in doubt; one chapter in this book described the development and testing of systematic approaches to collecting pressure ulcer prevalence data across several European countries. This initiative may assist with questions related to prevalence measures, but is prevalence the most appropriate form of audit we could adopt? Most would argue for pressure ulcer incidence or incidents to be reported; the challenge is how should this information be collected? If we do not accept and meet this challenge now then we will remain in ignorance regarding whether our efforts to tackle pressure ulceration have been ultimately successful. We would argue that this is not an acceptable scenario and that it is now time for pressure ulcer monitoring to come of age and demonstrate a maturity that can only come from the performance of systematic audits following nationally agreed methods.

One final challenge remains and it is by far the most embarrassing for those involved in pressure ulcers. Have we, through all our research, our focus on practice, the development of a strong commercial sector supporting pressure ulcer care and the production of publications such as this, had any demonstrable effect on the number of people affected each year with pressure ulcers. We may all individually think we know the answer to this question but no formal data exists to indicate that fewer people develop pressure ulcers today compared with ten years ago. If we are truly to move the pressure ulcer debate forward, we cannot afford not to be able to answer this question. That is why this book began with sections on pressure ulcer epidemiology, the need for consistent recording of data and the overriding requirement that such data be truly comparable.

Michael Clark
Senior Research Fellow
Wound Healing Research Unit
University of Wales College of Medicine, Cardiff
February, 2004

Final note

Since the early 1990s when the Department of Health (United Kingdom) set the first national challenge, 'to reduce the incidence of pressure ulcers by 5%–10% per annum', and pressure ulcers became a marker of quality in healthcare, much has been achieved. Evidence reviews have been published, national and European prevention and treatment guidelines have been developed and, as this book illustrates, research continues across the spectrum; from the microcellular to the organisational level. Yet, despite these initiatives, epidemiological studies still report overall prevalence levels that are not too disimilar from those of fifteen years ago and, while the severity of the wounds may have declined over time, most healthcare providers continue to encounter individuals with grade 3 or 4 tissue damage.

Recent trends (2003–4), within the United Kingdom, would indicate that we are about to witness a renewed wave of interest in pressure ulcers. During 2003, the inspectorate for the Commission for Health Improvement increasingly published pressure ulcer rates within their summary statement, while the National Health Service Litigation Authority recognises the benefit of having a comprehensive, and audited, pressure ulcer policy. The latest, and perhaps most radical change, is the emergent practice of reporting pressure ulcer development as an 'adverse clinical event'. This change of approach falls under the tenet of the National Patient Safety Agency whereby 'avoidable' incidents are fully investigated, not to lay blame, but rather to learn from the process and adopt strategies to reduce the risk of recurrence. With the National Institute of Clinical Excellence's pressure ulcer guidelines (2003) now providing recommendations for nurse training, clinical audit and patient involvement, we truly enter interesting times ahead. Once again, pressure ulcers are back under the spotlight, not only as a quality measure, but also as a measure of patient safety and well-being.

References

DoH (1992) *The Health of the Nation: A Strategy for Health in England*. HMSO, London
NICE (2003) *Pressure Ulcer Prevention*. NICE, London

Lyn Phillips
Clinical and Communications Manager
Huntleigh Healthcare Limited
March, 2004

Huntleigh Healthcare Limited has devoted thirty years to research and development in this field. We are proud to work in partnership with experts, not only to provide state of the art solutions but also to support educational initiatives such as this book. Making a difference through knowledge.

List of acknowledgements

The authors of *Chapter 4* would like to thank:

Mr Kawasato and Ms Kodomari for their technical assistance. This work was supported in part by a Grant for Scientific Research from the Japanese Ministry of Education, Science and Culture (project number: C-09672407).

Iain Swain (*Chapter 5*) would like to thank:

Cheryl Dunford, Peter Stacey and Ellis Peters for all their hard work on the Department of Health trial as well as the Medical Devices Agency for the funding of this work. He would also like to thank Diane Norman, Steve Morant and Wendy Wareham for all the consultancy work that they have undertaken over the past ten years. Without all of their efforts the data would not have been available to write this paper.

Dan Bader (*Chapter 5*) would like to acknowledge the support of many collaborators, including:

Kath Bogie, George Cochrane, Isaac Nuseibeh and Carlijn Bouten. The latter helped the development of the experimental model to examine the effects of pressure and time in the onset of cellular damage.

Index